The International Library

THE PSYCHOLOGY OF
SPECIAL ABILITIES AND
DISABILITIES

Founded by C. K. Ogden

The International Library of Psychology

DEVELOPMENTAL PSYCHOLOGY
In 32 Volumes

are found.   But there is also great value in discovering abilities which exist and in endeavoring to base constructive measures on them.

It is fully recognized that many of the questions concerning special abilities and disabilities cannot yet be solved.   It is hoped, however, that the present discussion will lead to appreciation of the need for greater study in this field and will stimulate other efforts in this direction.

The whole presentation of the subject is based on the experience that many case-studies have afforded.   In the selection of cases, in the analysis of the material, and, indeed, in the preparation of the entire book I have been greatly helped by Doctor William Healy, to whom I gratefully acknowledge my indebtedness for inspiration, encouragement, and wise counsel.

AUGUSTA F. BRONNER.

CHICAGO,
    October, 1916.

PREFACE

WITH the ever increasing demand in education for recognition of the individual rather than the mass, it is remarkable that no attempt has been made as yet to formulate specifically the problems of specialized abilities and disabilities. On the side of mental defect, interest is centered so largely on testing and caring for individuals of general low intelligence that the problems of narrower types of defect have been neglected and still are largely misunderstood. Some writers have touched upon related questions, mainly in referring to the fact of individual differences in mental capacities, but only general statements are to be found ; nowhere else have special defects been outlined and nowhere can one find even enumeration of the types of variation that are practically important.

In this book an attempt has been made to discuss practical aspects of special abilities and disabilities, to offer in detail methods of attacking problem-cases, and to present various types, both (*a*) of particular disabilities in those who have normal general ability and (*b*) of particular abilities in those who are below normal in general capacities. The great tendency of to-day in the psychological study of individuals is to make general diagnoses, stressing particularly the defects that

First published in 1917 by
Routledge
2 Park Square, Milton Park, Abingdon, Oxfordshire OX14 4RN
711 Third Avenue, New York, NY 10017

First issued in paperback 2014

Routledge is an imprint of the Taylor and Francis Group, an informa business

British Library Cataloguing in Publication Data
A CIP catalogue record for this book
is available from the British Library

The Psychology of Special Abilities and Disabilities
ISBN 0415-20983-8
Developmental Psychology: 32 Volumes
ISBN 0415-21128-X
The International Library of Psychology: 204 Volumes
ISBN 0415-19132-7

ISBN 13: 978-1-138-87510-4 (pbk)
ISBN 13: 978-0-415-20983-0 (hbk)

THE PSYCHOLOGY OF SPECIAL ABILITIES AND DISABILITIES

AUGUSTA F BRONNER

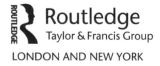

Routledge
Taylor & Francis Group

LONDON AND NEW YORK

CONTENTS

THE PSYCHOLOGY OF SPECIAL ABILITIES AND DISABILITIES

CHAPTER I

THE PROBLEM

THAT human beings have particular abilities and disabilities varying more or less — and frequently varying greatly — from the level of normal capacity, is a fact of much psychological interest as well as of great practical educational and social significance. In recent years psychologists have concerned themselves quite as much with individual differences as with the formulation of general laws. They have been interested in the variabilities that exist in any group, as well as in the common trends that are shown. They have laid down the general principle that all men differ in all traits. Thorndike has stated again and again that there is no "typical mind"; that differences exist at birth and increase with progress toward maturity. "Individuality is already clearly manifest in children of school age. The same situation evokes widely differing responses; the same task is done

1

at differing speeds and with different degrees of success; the same treatment produces differing results." [1]

Experimental studies of different mental processes have led to the conclusion that, in all of their abilities, the majority of individuals cluster about an average; the greater the divergence from the average, the smaller the number of individuals found. One practical corollary of this general truth is, that while most people can adjust themselves satisfactorily to ordinary situations, there are some so far removed from the average that they are ill-adjusted under these same circumstances. It is to these persons, numerically in the minority, yet forming a class socially very significant, that injustice is done in the present state of affairs. It is they who are often misunderstood, neglected, allowed to remain with their best possibilities undeveloped. It is for them, the individuals with particular abilities and disabilities, we would bespeak intelligent consideration. Among educators the most discerning thinkers have recognized this group as one meriting special consideration. "The cry for individual adjustment has become a shibboleth among the reformers," says Suzzallo, but, alas, the cry has met little response in action.

Only when variations are extreme have they been recognized; the organization of special classes and institutions for the crippled, the deaf, the blind, the feeble-minded, and the epileptic, has been a step in the right direction. However, this will not suffice; variations less obvious, but equally as significant, can no longer be entirely disregarded. To classify all persons into groups of the normal or the defective is altogether inadequate for the purposes of education and other social adjustments. Yet, at present, this is exactly what is almost universally done. Children are placed either in groups of the normal and taught

[1] Thorndike, E. L., "Individuality", 1911.

accordingly, or are placed in special classes for defectives and taught by methods supposedly adapted to their given type. But, if there are particular abilities and disabilities in various mental traits, no such division of method will suffice to educate all in the best way.

Study of the correlations that exist between different mental traits is another field of experimentation that bears upon our problem. These studies, made by Spearman,[1] by Pearson,[2] Burt,[3] Thorndike,[4] and others, have shown that the possession of ability in one direction increases the probability of possessing ability in other directions. But correlations are far from perfect, and no one denies that in some cases superiority in one trait may be accompanied by actual incapacity or specialized defect in other traits. Hence the statement that in general correlations in mental life are positive offers no criticism to the finding of special abilities and special defects. Indeed, such findings are quite in accord with those laws of mental life which are at present known.

That many facts concerning mental life have not yet been discovered will be readily conceded. One contribution that the study of problem-cases will no doubt make is to the better understanding of the normal functioning of mental processes. It has been largely through the study of pathological conditions that knowledge of physiology has been increased. The observation of results following disease, injury, or defects of special parts of the central nervous system, has been one of the chief means of

[1] Spearman and Krueger, "Die Korrelation zwischen verschiedenen geistigen Leistungsfähigkeiten." *Zeitschrift für Psychologie*, 44, 1906.
[2] Pearson, K., "On the Relationship of Intelligence to Size and Shape of Head and to Other Physical and Mental Characters." *Biometrika*, 5, 1907.
[3] Burt, Cyril, "Experimental Tests of General Intelligence." *British Journal of Psychology*, 3, 1909.
[4] Thorndike, E. L., "Heredity, Correlation and Sex Differences in School Abilities." "Columbia University Contributions to Philosophy", etc., XI, 1903.

gaining knowledge about its structure and functioning. Perhaps analogous methods might prove as valuable in the understanding of psychological problems, for much is yet to be learned of the processes underlying complex mental activities. Until laws concerning the processes involved in actual performance have been scientifically established, individual adjustments cannot be made rationally and successfully.

Let us see how inadequately the problem of individual adjustment is being met at the present time, first, from the point of view of the school. According to our present practice, the child enters school without his particular characteristics or idiosyncrasies being known to the teacher. Nowhere is opportunity offered for any definite study of the individual, and except as peculiarities and variations from the rest of the class are so extreme as to attract attention, differences among members of the group remain unknown. Of course, obvious traits are learned as time goes on, but the recognition of even these depends on the astuteness of the teacher, her interest in the pupils, her powers of observation and judgment. That such subjective standards are inaccurate, often false, we know by experimental studies which have been made where judgments of various teachers in regard to the same pupil are found to vary greatly.

Certain it is that the more subtle characteristics, which often are most important practically, remain unknown. Comments regarding character, mental make-up, unusual traits are rarely made, and when made, are not always considered worth recording. The next year the class passes on to another teacher; whatever information had been garnered previously is lost; all that is usually noted is the achievement in the different school subjects in terms of a scale of numbers or letters whose values are determined arbitrarily, according to each individual teacher's subjective standard. Usually not a word is appended concerning the dozen and one observations that even the most obtuse teacher must have made of each individual child, though these might save weeks or even months of maladjustment for the child and confusion and misunderstanding on the part of the next teacher. What a waste of knowledge gained through the daily experience of a whole school year!

If it were practicable to have each child studied in such a way as to reveal his best possibilities and talents, that is, if there were scientific educational diagnoses, it is quite conceivable that much more might be accomplished even with bright children than is now the case. And where there has not been obvious failure, we do not know how much greater success might have been achieved under circumstances more favorable to the individual's development. As conditions now are, some children learn because they are fortunate enough to receive good training; no doubt many more learn in spite of poor training, or, at least, training not adapted to their individual needs; others, because of unrecognized innate peculiarities, do not progress satisfactorily at all.

Every teacher knows the child who merely drags along, yet seems in general fairly bright. Then, there is the child who does very well in some subjects, but who is exceedingly retarded in others. Procedure in regard to these children varies; in some schools, when a child is a failure in some one school subject, he is pushed ahead in spite of this, with the consequence that in this subject he falls farther and farther behind the class. In other schools children are not promoted unless the results in *all* the school studies are satisfactory. In such cases the child fails of promotion again and again, although capable of advancing in some studies, with the dire effects that result from discouragement, from associating with younger children, and without even the compensation of being helped to master his difficulties.

We are not here considering the case of the generally stupid child who is an out-and-out school failure, who shows no ability in any one of the school subjects, who cannot maintain his position in the class. Such children have now the benefit of special classes, designated by various names. However, there is little recognition of the type of problem that we have in mind, and arrangements for meeting it are not at all common. In most instances the child is carried on in the class without even an understanding of the exact nature of the trouble.

The results of the present haphazard, irrational procedure are often serious; they lead to loss of interest in school work in general, to discouragement and feeling of inefficiency which frequently lie at the root of disciplinary problems. The step from this to truancy is easily made, and from that to more serious delinquency. Educational dissatisfaction is a very frequent beginning of what may develop into a long career of misdeeds. From our studies of delinquents we believe that misunderstanding and neglect of children with particular abilities and disabilities leads to truancy and thence to consequences the seriousness of which are too little appreciated.

We realize quite well that the school cannot be held responsible for all truancy that exists, that lack of home coöperation, bad companionship, and other forces may be causative factors. And yet, it would seem that if the school endeavored properly to meet its problems, it ought to be more of a restraining force and a more efficient competitor for the child's interest. It would be just as foolhardy to close our eyes to the fact that the school in and of itself must, in many cases, be the prime cause for truancy, as to adopt the opposite view, namely, that other forces are to blame altogether. Surely at least it behooves the school as a social agency to recognize this as one of the problems it must solve; to endeavor to make such a study as shall reveal the various factors involved; and, on the basis of these findings, intelligently to remedy blamable conditions.

Ordinary school methods, so lacking in individual adjustment, may explain too, in part, the vast retardation which exists. Again and again in our experience we have found children normal in the main, but who, nevertheless, are retarded two, three, or even more years in school. So many instances are found where other factors, physical ailments, social conditions, truancy, can be largely ruled out, that it seems only logical to account for retardation, in part, by present defects in schools. The regular curricula and methods are not achieving success in the case of children who have peculiarities which require special consideration.

Everywhere, in connection with this problem, common sense suggests the great waste that lack of appreciation of individual needs entails. There is the economic loss arising from school expenditures for efforts which accomplish little, but this is of slight consequence as compared with the waste of good human material, the making of truants and supposed dullards of those who might be developing useful talents.

Almost all that has been said in regard to the school situation is equally applicable to vocational life. The vocational misfit not only contributes poor work to society, but because of his inability to hold a job and his frequent changing from one place to another, he, too, often drifts into delinquency. There is, thus, loss to the public, to the employer, and to the employé. Vocational dissatisfactions are as frequent and quite as serious as educational maladjustments.

The problems we are here concerned with are, then,

those that arise because of lack of recognition of special
abilities and special disabilities — problems even outlined, so far as we know, only by Healy.[1] There is, on
the one hand, the individual who is normal except for
special mental defects, and, on the other, the individual
who, though in general mentally below normal, has some
special ability, which, if developed, might be highly significant for his future welfare. (It can at once be seen that
we are not dealing with the normal individual endowed
with unusual ability, the genius or supernormal; this is not
our problem, though the method used in the study of our
problem-cases and later explained in detail is equally
applicable for the study of the supernormal.)

Just what do we mean by the term "the individual
with special mental defect"? We mean a person with
some mental defect who could not rightfully be designated
feeble-minded, or even subnormal; one who proves by
tests and social reactions that, in the main, he is normal.
So-called general intelligence tests — Binet or other
"measuring scales of intelligence" — show, in these
cases, that the individual is not generally incapable, although results on certain tests and certain aspects of
behavior are not in accord with the general findings.
The extent of the incapacity may be more or less narrow.
Thus, it is conceivable that a person is defective in all
memory processes, or that he is normal, let us say, in
his visual memory, but decidedly poor in auditory
memory, or even that his disability lies in some very
narrow sphere of memory, perhaps for numbers only.
Obviously it is unfair and of no practical value to call such
a person feeble-minded or a "mental defective."

The individual mentally below normal in general, but
with special abilities, presents the reverse of this picture.
Of course, this group might include all grades of mental

<hr>

[1] Healy, William, "The Individual Delinquent", 1915.

defect where contrasted special ability exists. However, we are not now interested in discussing the so-called "idiot-savants", those rare individuals who, in spite of extreme amentia, show remarkable skill in some one direction. Their general intelligence is so limited that they are unable to adapt themselves to living conditions outside of institutions. Nor are we concerned with the feeble-minded of any grade possessing special abilities which cannot enable them to meet successfully ordinary social demands. But there are those who fall somewhat below the upper limits of feeble-mindedness (the Binet tests for the twelve-year level) according to the definition of the American Association for the Study of the Feeble-minded, and who yet possess abilities which, not discovered by these tests, render them able to compete in an ordinary environment. Then, there remains a group, by Healy called the subnormal, of those who, while definitely lacking in the higher mental powers as estimated by tests, yet pass the Binet twelve-year level and possess special abilities of social significance. It is these two latter classes that we have in mind in our discussion of defective individuals with special abilities.[1]

No doubt, many a person somewhat defective mentally is performing satisfactorily some type of lowly work, and

---

[1] It is interesting in this connection to note that neither of these last two groups conforms to the now widely accepted definition of feeble-mindedness formulated in accordance with social implications. The British Royal Commission for the Study of the Feeble-minded in 1908 defined the feeble-minded person as one who, suffering from incomplete cerebral development, is unable to perform his duties as a member of society in the position to which he was born. The remarkable new Illinois statute, framed in 1915, giving legal power of commitment of the feeble-minded, states that the criterion of feeble-mindedness in an individual is mental defect of a degree rendering him incapable of managing himself and his affairs. This would indicate that in spite of possible failure on psychological tests, the person who, for one reason or another, is able to care for himself and to succeed among his fellow men from an economic and moral standpoint, cannot properly be designated as feeble-minded.

many more could be educated to be economically independent and useful if special abilities were sought and trained. It is here the world at large is in great need of further study of defective individuals not segregated in institutions. In spite of much discussion and the formulation of many generalizations in regard to the feeble-minded, certain aspects of the question are rarely taken into account. At present, one great need is follow-up work in connection with this type, in order that we may know how many succeed in the world and why they are successful. Studies such as that made by Weidensall, who found in a group of successful maids a number feeble-minded as gauged by the Binet scale, need to be multiplied. Comparative studies of groups of individuals engaged in various types of occupations are now being undertaken and will, no doubt, be of great value in aiding us to reach safer conclusions regarding the relationship of mental defect and industrial capacity.

· Although the problem of the out-and-out defective, the feeble-minded, has been very widely discussed, that of the individual with special defect and the subnormal with special ability is largely neglected. But from the standpoint of social economy, of possible constructive measures, the problem of special abilities and disabilities is exceedingly important. We do not wish to minimize the social significance of the feeble-minded, involving the protection of the individual and of society. But in the case of individuals with special defect or special aptitude, it is a question of positive rather than of negative values, the contributing to society of something worth while. Their problem is not that of segregation; it is, rather, adjustment to the social organism.

To effect the best possible adjustment of any individual to the group, many concrete issues must be taken into account. In the cases where unusual conditions obtain, such as those found in the types with which we are here concerned, questions of etiology and certain medical problems as well as some social conditions are to be ever thought of in efforts at practical solutions. However, in the following chapters, the discussion of individual adjustments will be limited to educational and vocational considerations, omitting all else.

CHAPTER II

METHODS OF DIAGNOSIS

CERTAIN theoretical aspects of the problems concerning special abilities and special disabilities are of considerable interest. They deal with the question of the relations found between different mental traits in the same individual, including the degree of correlation between one mental function and another, and the proof of the presence or absence of mental compensations. Some psychologists believe that defects in certain fields are compensated by unusual excellence in other fields, a theory that has been held on the basis of extreme cases, as for example, the blind, who after losing sight show great skill in other sensory fields. The opponents of this point of view have, of course, interpreted such instances as evidence only of the effect of intensive training made necessary through lack of some sensory functions.

Another point of interest is the theoretical problem whether "all branches of intellectual activity have in common one fundamental function (or group of functions)" — a view held by Spearman and his followers. The opposite doctrine, namely, that given elements in different mental functions may be only loosely correlated, has been enunciated by Thorndike, who believes that "measurements reveal a high degree of independence of different mental functions even where to the abstract psychological theorist they have seemed nearly identical."

According to the latter view, one might expect to find special defect or unusual ability in any one of the mental processes. These processes, according to all psychologists, include sensation, perception, apperception, imagination, memory, association, judgment, and reasoning, as well as the emotions and will, the latter involving inhibition and initiative. To this list must be added the processes concerned with motor reactions.

Or we can think of our problem in terms of reactions which in themselves involve various combinations of the above mental processes. From this viewpoint we can study ability in the realms of number work, language, reading, spelling, handwork, and the other school subjects. Then, too, there is the whole question of complex functions, such as foresight and general powers of self-control. We might, also, consider the problem of the speed of mental processes and reactions rather than the character of the product.

In other words, if the mind represents a multitude of functions, we might expect to find defect or exceptional ability existing in any one function or in activities involving various combinations of functions. To study an individual thoroughly would involve knowing not only all his particular acquirements, but all the possibilities and potentialities that exist in highly specialized fields. Of course, this is an ideal that we can scarcely hope to attain; nor is it necessary, perhaps, for practical purposes. Interesting as all theoretical questions are, we wish, in reality, to know the defects that are stumbling blocks in the individual's career, and to discover abilities that may be practically utilized. This would be the great step forward.

To meet these issues intelligently there must be intensive study of each problem individual. For school purposes as well as for social and vocational adjustments it would hardly suffice to base educational methods upon the teacher's judgment or upon class standing, for the former, we know, is often somewhat inaccurate, and the latter tells merely the subjects in which the pupil fails or excels, nothing as to the cause of the failure or as to the possible existence of unused talents. This is no reflection upon the teacher, for it would be impossible to determine these significant points without analyzing school activities and studying the mental processes which underlie them.

What means can be employed in the study of the mental processes involved in various activities which will reveal facts significant for the explanation of individual differences in abilities? Psychological tests are now quite widely used for the study of mentality, the commonest procedure being the study of the individual by means of some "measuring scale." The best known of these is the Binet-Simon scale for measuring intelligence, or some adaptation or revision of this, such as Goddard's, Terman and Childs'; and Kuhlmann's. The purpose of these scales is the exploration of the individual's general intelligence, the estimation of ability in terms of age-levels whereby the individual can be diagnosed as normal in ability or retarded. In case the latter is true, the amount of retardation determines whether or not the individual is feeble-minded.

I shall not here enter into any criticism regarding these tests, for their inadequacies have already been so widely discussed. A "measuring scale" of intelligence gives a convenient starting point for the study of individuals and has certain other values. It is in such general use that it offers a convenient method for the comparison of the same individual by different persons; the age-level principle on which tests are based is an excellent one in some ways; the form in which results are stated is convenient if not altogether accurate. However, from the present point of view, it is sufficient to state that the mental functions tested thereby are, in general, quite similar, and for this very reason none of the scales now available is suited to our purpose. None includes tests for a wide range of different functions; indeed, many mental functions are not tested at all, and thus we are given very few clues to particular abilities or disabilities. While it is of great value to gauge a person's general intelligence — if there is such a thing — and to place him on a scale as compared to other individuals, yet this throws but little light upon the problems we are here discussing. Whatever the value of any such given system, it would seem that it must be supplemented by a wide range of other tests if one would make careful studies upon which to base prognoses and recommendations for practical guidance.

There are now many other tests available for the study of various mental processes, many more than can be here discussed; the number is almost legion, and new ones are being devised rapidly. With the means now at hand a fairly wide range of capacities can be studied. I shall simply mention some which we know by experience are valuable for practical purposes and which have been used in the study of problem cases later presented.

For determining an individual's success in solving problems involving concrete material many tests are now in use. The simplest of these are the so-called Form Boards, where the subject has only to distinguish between one form and another; there are the Dearborn and the Healy-Fernald construction tests; the so-called Puzzle Boxes; some of the Knox tests; the Stenquist test for mechanical ability, and many others, for which norms are being established and which either are or soon will be ready for general use.

Such performance tests with concrete material afford a means of evaluating the individual's ability in perception of form and form relationships. Further, they enable one to gauge the subject's method of attacking a problem; for instance, the test may be solved by random trial and error method, or by procedure which the individual plans. One of the most illuminating features is noting whether the subject profits by experience, whether he avoids or repeats impossibilities and unsuccessful efforts. The improvement made on later retrials gives an indication of learning ability in relation to a particular kind of situation. Any differences which may be found in readiness of learning, where the problems are presented thus concretely as opposed to problems presented in abstract form, become very significant from the standpoint of educational method. Our present-day practice still emphasizes very largely the acquiring of knowledge through abstract means, and rarely is this preceded by actual experience from which concepts and abstractions are in reality derived.

Aside from such study of the perceptual processes as are required in dealing with the above-mentioned problems, many other means are available for testing perception. Thus, we can gauge perception of color as well as of form, and ability to perceive differences between various forms; that is, to discriminate one form from another. For the latter purpose, the well-known cancellation tests may be used and others based upon the same principle. Perceptions in the abstract field involve mental traits which will be discussed under the reasoning process. In practical problems it is frequently necessary to study the individual's powers of perception with different kinds of material, as, for instance, with auditory or visual stimuli. For testing the former there have been devised elaborate instruments which are used in many laboratories. But quite as valuable for ordinary purposes are the rather rough, but sufficiently diagnostic ordinary speech tests, such as the repeating of phrases or stanzas which require good discrimination of sound.

Other tests are especially adapted to study the powers of apperception. The ability to size up a situation and to grasp the general meaning of it is exceedingly important in all activities of life, beginning earlier than the school age and extending long past it. Here is involved the relation of one part to another; perception in the light of something which has gone before. Such tests are possible for the apperception of ideas expressed in pictorial form, as in the Healy Pictorial Completion test, and of ideas expressed in words, as in the Ebbinghaus Mutilated Text. The work of Trabue in arranging a scale for the determination of apperception of ideas as expressed through the medium of written language will no doubt have a great value in such places as it is applicable.

The importance of memory in all the activities of life is so obvious that we need not dwell upon it. It is less commonly recognized, however, that memory itself is not a functional unit; it would be more accurate to speak of "memories", since the ability to remember in one field and by one avenue of approach is not always closely correlated with memory power in other fields. On the basis of actual study of individuals, it is frequently found that good memory for rote material does not necessarily mean equally good memory for logical material. Even in rote memory there are often specializations, for the span for auditory presentations may be quite different from that for visual presentations. No doubt it is true that there are differences in other specialized forms of memory, such as the motor and kinæsthetic, but for the practical purposes of educational training the above mentioned probably constitute the main fields for experimentation. We must distinguish, too, between tests for immediate and remote memory, the former, of course, implying a reproduction that immediately follows the stimulus, whatever that may be, and the latter a reproduction that follows after intervals that vary according to the wish of the experimenter.

Tests for memory span may consist of numerals or nonsense syllables presented either by auditory or visual means. Sometimes lists of related or unrelated words are used, whereas, for testing logical memory, a passage in which the ideas are logically related is used. Experiments in the field of memory have shown that there is, in general, a high correlation for various phases of the memory process, but it is unfortunately true that exceptions to this in individual cases are frequently found. It is just such exceptional cases that are often school and vocational problems.

Other tests are especially adapted to study processes, of association, either the control of old associations or the ability to form new ones. For the former there is the free association test, in which one association calls up another without any controlled relationship, or the well known Kent-Rosanoff test in which the subject reacts by giving the first word which the stimulus-word suggests. In the Woodworth-Wells association tests a stimulus is given, to which the subject reacts according to some principle which has been told him; he gives either the opposite of a word or a superordinate, or a word which stands in some other particular relationship to the stimulus word. These tests have been very widely used in the study of various psychoses, but are important in all studies of mentality, for they give a clue to the speed as well as to the accuracy of the association processes.

As for reasoning ability, here again we must remember we are not dealing with a unitary process. Reasoning is a complex activity in which a number of mental processes are involved; thus, the ability to form mental representations, to analyze, to compare, to form judgments, all are elements. Likewise one may be able to reason very well in certain realms and fail altogether in others. This is true, aside from the question of having acquired such knowledge or data as are necessary in order to reason at all. There are certain tests for the purpose of studying the separate elements which enter into the reasoning processes and still others intended to test reasoning as a whole in its relation to diverse situations. Some of the Binet tests deal with reasoning; Bonser [1] has offered a number of tests, all of which deal with reasoning, though the material itself is quite varied. Terman's tests for ingenuity, incorporated in his intelligence scale, require reasoning.

Turning for a moment to tests for the different psychological processes which are factors in reasoning, we find that for study of powers of mental representation there are the well known Cross Line and Code tests, which involve analysis and to some extent other functions as well, since visual or motor imagery may play quite a rôle. Ability to determine mentally similarities and differences is required in some of the Binet tests, where remembered objects are to be compared, and in tests included in the Terman revision. Tests for judgment vary greatly, since the situations requiring this mental process are of all kinds and descriptions. Thus, included in the Binet series are some very simple tests requiring judgment in the sensory fields. We must remember, of course, that incidental to many tests one can determine the subject's ability to judge.

For studying the powers of psychomotor control there are the tests requiring apparatus, such as the " 3-hole

[1] Bonser, F. G., "Reasoning Ability of Children ", "Teachers College Contributions to Education ", 37, 1910.

test", where the task is to hold a stylus without touching
the sides of the hole in which it is inserted; or, there are
simpler tests, such as drawing a line between two given
lines without touching the edges, or placing a dot in
half-inch squares as rapidly as possible without touching the lines or missing the squares. These tests for
psycho-motor control, or motor coördination, may be
supplemented by other tests commonly used by neurologists.

Mental control may be evaluated by results achieved
on quite a varied group of tests, including the association
tests, already mentioned, and the Kraepelin Continuous
Addition and Subtraction tests, where a certain number
must be added or subtracted continuously from some
given starting point. Here, both speed and accuracy
are significant. Some of the Rossolimo tests, such as
naming the months backward, or obeying several commands simultaneously, are designed for this same
purpose.

We can only mention briefly a few other tests which
are practically useful in diagnosing abilities. Among
these, one interesting and important group of tests is
designed to determine the subject's ability to follow directions. Obeying commands, as in the seven-year Binet
test, offers the simplest form, while the Instruction Box
and the Knox Cube test present problems concerned with
tasks involving concrete material, and the Woodworth-
Wells Direction tests, for the same purpose, present the
directions in printed form. Important also is another
group of tests devised to show the individual's ability to
formulate generalizations on the basis of repeated experience, as in the so-called Multiple Choice Test, one important and practically useful form of which has recently
been devised by Yerkes.

Incidental to all testing, there is opportunity for observing power of attention and distractability, qualities which can be gauged also by specific tests for this purpose. Characteristic traits such as persistence and determination, as opposed to easy discouragement, likewise may be noted.

Concerning the emotions, the affective side of life, few tests are as yet in use, though most students of behavior appreciate the need for them. Indeed, it is quite doubtful if tests will ever offer an effective means of studying these complex aspects of mentality. The situations which in real life call the emotions into play are not easily duplicated in the laboratory, and artificial stimuli for arousing them necessarily would result in totally different reactions. How can one study experimentally love and hate as they affect behavior? Or what can tests reveal concerning the formation and results of anti-social grudges? Judgment as to defects in emotional life, as well as in regard to will, must be based very largely if not altogether upon the individual's social reactions. Recognition of individual differences in strength of the emotions, in powers of inhibition and self-control, will probably always rest mainly upon evidence gleaned from general behavior and incidental reactions rather than upon results obtained by use of one psychological test or series of tests.

As for the school subjects, we can, of course, determine more or less accurately the results that have accrued from the years spent in the schoolroom. Where failure to profit by educational opportunities is due to real defect, it becomes essential to study the processes involved. Although the psychology of the school subjects is as yet largely unknown, and, as we have already stated, this limits the possibility of reaching a satisfactory explanation of all instances of school failures, yet one must go as far as is possible in an effort to find the causes upon which alone remedial measures can be undertaken. We shall discuss these questions more fully as problems of various kinds are presented.[1]

Of course, intensive study by means of a wide range of tests requires a great amount of time. The more thorough the study and the more one endeavors to make a complete survey of the individual's capacities in various directions, the more time is needed. But the value of the findings and the accuracy of the results are in direct proportion to the time expended. Then, too, the clinical psychologist must be familiar with a wide range of tests, and in certain instances must have sufficient ingenuity to adapt means to the problem in hand.

Furthermore, he must have the ability to analyze the results, since often it is not sufficient merely to compare findings with established norms; it is even more necessary to interpret divergences. The ideal diagnostician would, no doubt, be difficult to find, since medical and neurological training, general psychological knowledge, and experience in clinical psychology ought to be supplemented by experience in the educational field. We can only hope to approximate this ideal. We can, at least, demand a person who has had fairly wide training and experience, who realizes the various aspects which may be conditioning factors, and who supplements his own knowledge by consulting others who can add the facts needed to make well-rounded studies possible.

[1] Such a book as Freeman's "Experimental Education" (1916) gives only a partial analysis of the school subjects, and while suggestive and helpful, it does not offer much practical help in the solution of problem cases.

CHAPTER III

DIFFERENTIAL DIAGNOSIS

IN the preceding chapter we have discussed the possibility of studying in detail the various mental processes in their relationship to the capabilities of the individual. However, before there can be a final diagnosis upon which to base practical procedure, certain interpretative considerations must be weighed. The psychological examination is not sufficient in and of itself to enable one to reach a diagnosis; rather, here, as in medicine, we need differential diagnosis. This means a much broader acquaintance with the problems of psychopathology than mere familiarity with tests indicates. Abnormal reactions to tests are outward signs that require interpretation, since they may be due to any one of a number of causes. Hence, the various possibilities must be known and considered before concluding that we have a case of either general mental defect or special mental disability.

Here should be emphasized the fact that data must be gathered from various sources in order to make an intelligent study of an individual. Even for educational diagnosis much more is needed than the findings obtained from psychological tests. Adequate case-studies here, as in other problems, require a knowledge of the conditions in the background, including data concerning heredity, family history, developmental history and environmental conditions. One can intelligently understand an individual only in the light of all these facts.

23

Differential diagnosis of special ability hardly needs discussion since any unusual capacity in a special field is a positive fact needing no further interpretation. In both normal individuals and defectives it is necessary to test the different mental functions in order that where special abilities exist they may be brought to light. The only generalization that needs emphasis is that in order to discover special gifts there must be a search for them. That is, a wide enough range of tests must be used to give each individual a chance to display his capacities. Once discovered, there should follow a proper evaluation of abilities, as is not commonly done, for it is the part of common sense to utilize for the benefit of the individual and society such gifts as exist.

Differential diagnosis of special defects is a much more complex problem, since, in general, negative results may be due to exceedingly varied causes. Irregularity in test results, which, on superficial view, might seem indicative of special defect, may, for example, be due instead to *poor physical conditions*. This necessitates a physical examination in the case of every individual who is studied.   Physical disability preventing the best achievement of which one is capable may be reflected in work in the laboratory where mental examinations are made, in the schoolroom, or in the shop.

Interest and zest for mental pursuits is sometimes maintained in spite of poor physical background, we know; such studies as those of Gulick and Ayres [1] have shown this. Nevertheless, it is not true in all cases. We ourselves know instances where, with improved health, the reports on conduct and school standing, and also the industrial record, were greatly changed. We know, too, cases where findings on tests were altogether

[1] Gulick and Ayres, "Medical Inspection of Schools", Chapter XII, 1908.

different after the child had been built up physically. Anemia, malnutrition, or debility following illness, is sometimes the explanation of mental dullness which might be confused with innate defect. In all such cases it seems only fair to give the individual the benefit of the doubt. He needs, in any case, all the physical help which can be given him, and unless the mental disability is so extreme as to preclude any possibility of poor physical conditions as an explanation, the final diagnosis should be held in abeyance. To be remembered always, particularly with young children, are the recently studied disturbances of function of the glands of internal secretion. Both we and many others have seen results nothing short of marvelous through treatment of these troubles in children who appeared exceedingly dull in some aspect of their mental life. This makes us all the more conscious of the contributions that future research may bring forth concerning relationships between physical and mental conditions.

Case 1. By way of illustration of the effect of physical conditions on mental life, we cite the case of Edith N., who represents findings that are not at all uncommon in our experience.[1] When twelve years old she was brought to the clinic by her mother. At that time she was in the fourth grade of the public school. We found her to be in very poor condition physically, suffering from anemia, defective vision, enlarged glands; there was a history of former otorrhea; the girl was dull and listless,

[1] The case-studies which are cited throughout are selected solely to illustrate the various types of abilities and disabilities, irrespective of age, sex, or nationality. That they include many more instances of males than females is probably due to the fact that in our clinic where court cases are largely studied, the number of males exceeds by far the number of females. Should any actual sex differences exist, they could only be determined on the basis of large numbers of unselected cases, a requirement which even our extensive material does not meet.

The detailed results of psychological examinations for each case will be found in the appendix.

and the results on psychological tests were very poor. According to Binet scale she ranged as 9⅔ years mentally. She failed on our simpler Construction Test and did very little in the way of school work, failing to spell correctly anything but the easiest words, or to solve any number work but the very simplest. The case was referred to a clinic for physical treatment and later to a convalescent home.

Thirteen months after this we had occasion to study this case once more. We found then that our advice had been acted upon, with the result that the girl had improved immensely. She had gained about twenty-six pounds in weight, had grown an inch; her vision was corrected by glasses, her throat was in good condition, tonsils and adenoids had been removed. Altogether she showed a wonderful improvement. The interesting feature from the point of view of our present discussion was the tremendous gain which we found on the mental side. She now passed up through the twelve-year Binet tests; solved correctly the Construction Test, which was previously a failure, as well as a more difficult one, which had not been tried before. A number of other tests corroborated these findings. We noted that she still was very poor in school work, but it must be remembered that during the intervening period she had practically no opportunity of attending school. Furthermore, she showed little interest in school; perhaps her discouragement was a natural state of affairs, since she was in a very low grade for a girl of her age. But it would be the height of folly to state that her school retardation was an evidence of innate mental defect, just as earlier it would have been altogether unfair not to have taken into account the effect of the poor physical conditions upon test results.

We may note that there are three general aspects to

the problem of the relation of physical disability to mental performance. First, poor physical conditions may not affect the quality of mental activities at all; second, psychological examination in the laboratory may not reveal the influence of poor physical status on mental achievement, particularly if the examination is brief and hence requires little prolonged attention and effort. But inability to cope with the requirements of school life may nevertheless be the direct result of the lack of physical vigor and health. Third, poor physical conditions may directly affect performance on tests as well as other mental effort.

It can readily be understood that in reaching a diagnosis of mental capacities one must be careful not to confuse innate disability with special defect due to a *defective sensory organ*. I need but mention troubles with vision and hearing. It requires hardly a moment's reflection to be convinced of the vast amount of routine school work that is profitless to a child who either cannot see or hear normally. It is quite generally recognized that sensory defects frequently act as irritants, influencing a wider range of activity than those correlated with the actual sense organ itself. Eye strain coupled with visual defect leads to nervousness and irritability; the consequences of several types of ear troubles, such as variability of hearing that accompanies otorrhea, are equally important. Many a child is accounted stupid who is really dull from remediable sensory defects. Much as these subjects have been discussed, we find many instances where there has been utter neglect of such troubles. In spite of our present method of medical inspection in schools, there are, we know from experience, many cases of children who have unrecognized physical ailments which affect their school work to an extent that is altogether unappreciated.

Case 2. Recently a nine-year old boy was brought to us because, on the basis of supposed defect for school work, he was believed to be a suitable subject for the state institution for the feeble-minded. He had attended school for three years and was still in the first grade. He was indeed dull looking, and had one dared form an impression from his appearance and listless manner, one might have concluded that the boy was mentally defective. Physical examination showed him to be virtually blind in one eye with vision about two thirds of normal in the other. He was a sufferer from chronic otorrhea, and when examined in the clinic he was found to be partially deaf. Inquiry regarding the school career elicited the fact that the boy had never been examined by the school physician, that no recognition had ever been made of the fact that he was suffering from sensory defects which required immediate attention. Psychological examination proved that the boy tested almost normal for his age.

Case 3. For similar reasons we studied a boy where the neglect of visual defect was equally egregious. He, too, was considered by his teachers as unable to learn school subjects, but a careful mental examination by us showed the boy was rather in advance of his chronological age, and was suffering from excessive visual defect. Sent to a correctional institution, he had broken his glasses shortly after commitment, and during the nine months which intervened between that time and our examination, his eyes had never been retested nor had glasses been obtained for him, and yet, in this case, the main reason for commitment was to give the lad educational opportunities.

So obvious is the distinction between special defect in the language field and poor results on tests due to *speech defect*, that we need but mention it. It is quite generally recognized that stuttering or stammering may retard normal progress as well as become a great factor in conduct problems. Of course, such defects can scarcely be overlooked in mental examination, and the only caution to be observed is a proper interpretation of the extent of the influence on both test results and school standing. Any diagnosis of mentality based solely on Binet or any "measuring scale", which consists largely of language tests, is altogether to be discountenanced in the study of individuals with speech defects.

Nervous disorders of one kind or another are, as one would expect, important influences in mental life, causing peculiarities which may lead to test results that can readily be confused with special defect, hence differential diagnosis here becomes of exceeding importance. This is notably true in cases of *hysteria* because of the reactions which characterize this nervous disease. Janet[1] and other authorities agree that in practically all cases of hysteria there is great variability in the functioning of the mental processes, that want of mental unity and deficiency of inhibition are essential features of the disorder. There is often extreme dissociation in the mental life and lack of control of both the emotions and of voluntary actions. The contradictory behavior to which this leads is a notable accompaniment of the disease. Frequently, too, there is simulation, so that the reactions of such persons are altogether unreliable.

These characteristic symptoms are such that when diagnosis of hysteria has been made, it becomes extremely dangerous to designate the individual as feeble-minded on the basis of tests. There are, indeed, two aspects that must be remembered in this problem. On the one hand, it is not contended by any authority that the diagnosis of hysteria can be made on the basis of mental tests alone,

[1] Janet, Pierre, "The Major Symptoms of Hysteria", 1907.

but, on the other hand, the best authorities would be equally as unwilling to state that mental tests are not directly affected by hysteria. Remembering the mental states of hystericals as described by Janet and others, it is to be expected that this disease will influence greatly the results of the psychological examination. The poor powers of control, together with definite inhibitions which sometimes occur, the dissociations and simulations, frequently, if not always, play a great rôle in the mental findings.

We ourselves have noted again and again the extraordinary variability in the mental processes that accompanies hysteria. Sometimes because of very definite attitude or simulation of one kind or another, the peculiarity may be evidenced on tests of one kind alone, in which case the differential diagnosis between this and specialized defect becomes very important.

Case 4. We might quote from our own experience the instance of a girl whom we studied at various times over an interval of two and a half years. She had been tested in several other laboratories, in one of which she was diagnosed as feeble-minded, a diagnosis made, no doubt, without any recognition of the fact that she was unmistakably a case of hysteria, and that therefore actual test results required interpretation in the light of this fact. Knowing the dangers inherent in such a situation, we were for long unwilling to make a definite statement regarding the girl's innate mental ability. Her reactions when first tested were significant because of their great irregularity. When seen some time later, we felt the psychological findings were still unreliable, owing to a distinctly bad attitude which the girl still assumed. Eventually, however, we had an opportunity of stimulating her powers of self-control, due to the fact that she herself knew her immediate future depended very largely on the outcome of the psychological examination, since the question was to be settled regarding her return to a correctional institution, her transfer to a school for the feeble-minded, or her living in a private home. Under these conditions we found that the girl was innately quite capable; that she could cope successfully with a number of difficult tests. Only where particularly good mental control was required were the results below normal. In their entirety, the test results were remarkably better than those found earlier by any one.

The irregular mental functioning of *chorea* must be interpreted in the light of the nervous disturbance. The findings on tests are often curiously bizarre and may lead to fallacious conclusions concerning special defect if the fact of the disease is not taken into account. Clinical psychologists should remember that in rare cases the only signs of chorea may be the mental disturbance and that some authorities contend that in every case mental functioning is at some time affected.

In differential diagnosis of special defect we must likewise consider the question of *epilepsy*, including the major and minor forms of the disease. All epileptologists unite in stating that mental peculiarities are found in as great or even greater measure in individuals subject to minor attacks as when convulsions occur. One of the notable peculiarities displayed by epileptics is the variability of their mental processes from day to day and in one field as compared to another. Very frequently the results on tests performed at one sitting are exceedingly irregular, and they may be found to vary considerably on retesting on another day. This is true apart from the fact that the mind is affected by actual epileptic attacks; not only is there variance in mental processes either immediately before or after a seizure, but in many instances the general variability of the epileptic's mental powers is equally characteristic at all times. When the careful investigation of developmental history that should always be made in cases of apparent special mental defect indicates the presence of epilepsy, test results must be interpreted in the light of this fact. It would be a very questionable procedure to reach a final diagnosis of the mentality of the epileptic on the basis of one examination, if results apparently showed defective powers. Of course, this is not equally true in instances where it is readily found that the epileptic individual is bright or normal mentally, as may frequently be the case.

Sometimes mental dullness caused by excessive use of *tea* or *coffee*, or by *smoking* indulged in to an extreme degree, exhibits itself in a form which makes observers suspicious of specialized defect. This is due to the fact that such habits may bring about lack of self-control, lack of interest, and inability to sustain attention. Hence, tasks which require persistent effort or continuity of purpose may be badly performed although there is no innate defect to account for this.

Case 5. We here may cite the case of a boy in the subnormal room of the public school who was accounted exceedingly dull by his teacher because, while he was able to do fairly well certain tasks which aroused his interest, yet he made little progress in abstract work. On psychological examination we found him to be exceedingly apathetic and unwilling to exert himself, frequently preferring to say that he could not do a test rather than to try. When stimulated to make an effort, he solved correctly problems which he had previously given up. We, too, noted the irregular test results, for he made quite a good record on performance tests which awakened his interest, but failed very frequently on tests of the *questionnaire* type. Naturally, this affected the Binet score markedly. Investigation of the family circumstances revealed the fact that there was extreme poverty, that several social agencies were supplying help, that the main article of the boy's diet was coffee, which he drank to excess. This was quite enough to account for both the nervous irritability, leading to bad conduct, and the mental apathy, leading to poor school work.

The relationship of *alcoholism* to mental disturbances which might be confused with special defect needs mention, though it should be added that very rarely does this problem present itself practically, because alcoholism in individuals young enough to be brought to the clinic is very infrequent. Although the number of such cases in our own experience has not been large, yet we have seen adolescents whose mental processes functioned most irregularly because of indulgence in alcohol. After the effect of this stimulant had worn off, the test results were quite different from what was obtained in earlier testing. The kind of irregularity found may vary from one case to another, exhibiting itself either in failure on tests which require good mental control, or on tests of some type which fail to awaken interest. Parenthetically, it may be interesting to mention that the selective effect of alcoholism is clearly seen in Korsakow's syndrome, where, temporarily at least, the individual loses certain powers, such as memory for recent events and orientation in time relationships.

In the enumeration of conditions which have caused mental irregularities that require differentiation from special defect, one of exceeding importance must be included, which, because often learned only through obtaining the child's confidence, is frequently entirely overlooked. I refer to the excessive indulgence in *bad sex practices* so commonly accompanied by extreme mental debility and causing results on tests that are often misinterpreted. It is a very interesting fact that such habits do not necessarily lead to general mental dullness so much as to lack of energy and mental apathy which shows itself in the inability to concentrate and maintain attention. For this reason tests which are rapidly completed are performed satisfactorily, in contradistinction to failure on work which requires continuity of purpose and steadiness of attention. Because of this, such cases may readily be confused with problems of true special defect. The retesting of such individuals is a matter of extreme interest, for we have noted again and again that with the conquering of bad habits there results great improvement on mental tasks.

Practically the only major *psychosis* that requires differentiation from special defect among adolescents is dementia præcox. Where other insanities occur, where there is melancholia or mania, the symptoms are so pronounced that there can be no doubt of the diagnosis. As for *dementia præcox*, how can it be distinguished from special defect? We know that this mental disease is characterized by lack of energy and diminution in the power of application; there is usually great torpidity and inattention, while the association processes are disturbed, especially from the standpoint of time reactions. But the individual's attitude toward the world in general is the main characteristic which leads to suspicion of aberration, and in this respect individuals suffering from dementia præcox are so unlike normal individuals with special defect that there is little likelihood of making an error if one keeps in mind the special traits which distinguish this psychosis. In this connection it must ever be remembered that mental aberration may affect test results to such an extent that it becomes impossible to determine how innately capable an individual really is. Diagnosis in regard to native capacity must, therefore, in such cases, be held in abeyance, or at least only tentatively stated.

Where severe *head injuries* have been received, leading to what is generally known as traumatic constitution, one may find peculiarities in the functioning of the mental processes which are somewhat similar to results due to special defect. The instability that arises from such injuries, lack of good powers of control and persistence, causes certain types of work to be badly performed.

Case 6. A boy who had suffered a severe head injury when nine years old was studied at our clinic, where it was found that the lad was extremely bright. He was now fifteen years of age, had reached eighth grade and was able to do well quite difficult school work. Later this boy was examined by a psychologist who diagnosed the case as one of feeble-mindedness, a conclusion based on Binet findings. In discussing several difficult tests which were performed very well, the opinion was rendered that these were merely evidences of narrowly specialized ability. The fact that this boy could do difficult problems in arithmetic by ingenious and economical methods, though he made a poor record on the Courtis tests which require long continued powers of attention, was not interpreted in the light of traumatic constitution, although this is a point of much importance. The difficult tasks which elicited interest and which could be rather quickly performed were done very well, although much more simple tests of the *questionnaire* type were failures. It was because of the poor record on such *questionnaire* and language tests that the boy was considered feeble-minded. The inconsistency between the failures on simple work and the successes on more difficult tasks should have made the experimenter seek explanation other than that of innate general defect.

Seen still later in our clinic, the test results were very

different from the last ones reported to us. Even by Binet tests no mental defect was found; the tests for upper years were done exceptionally well, as were, indeed, many other fairly difficult mental tasks. The explanation of these incontrovertible findings can only be the variations in mental functionings which are prone to occur, perhaps on the basis of emotional attitude, in cases of traumatic constitution.

We cannot here enter into a thorough discussion of the problem of the *constitutional inferior*. For details we refer the reader to the work of others, particularly to the informing discussion in Healy's "The Individual Delinquent." Suffice it for our purpose to state that constitutional inferiors present both physical and mental peculiarities, the latter of which cause test results that are quite variable and that require differentiation from special defect. Diagnosis in such cases can only be determined in the light of all the facts revealed by physical and psychological examination, as well as by family and developmental history and the story of the social career.

The clinical psychologist who wishes to be thorough and to diagnose intelligently must acquaint himself with these types. The same may be said in regard to certain other problems which can be understood only when much information besides that obtained from psychological examination is at hand. Thus, there are special defects which are due to brain injuries or to *disease of certain portions of the brain*. Aphasia, alexia, agraphia, word-deafness, and other such disturbances are, as defined by neurologists, always due to brain lesion and not to innate defect; they involve loss or impairment of power that once existed.

The problems of so-called congenital alexia, congenital word-blindness and word-deafness, we shall consider in detail in a later chapter. Suffice it to say here that in any case it requires care to distinguish between word-blindness and word-deafness due to cerebral lesions or defects, and symptoms similar in character, but due to grave difficulties with sight and hearing which at the time of examination may or may not have been corrected and which earlier were a severe handicap. (For further discussion of these points see Chapter VI.)

Certain considerations of *attitude* must ever be kept in mind in the diagnosis of mentality, because they have a very direct bearing upon the problem of differential diagnosis of special defect. Whatever affects attitude has a very vital relationship to all mental effort; as most important should be mentioned simulation and emotional disturbances. The attitude with which an individual approaches a task is a great factor in the results accomplished; fear, embarrassment, general depression, indeed, any emotion, may lead to most equivocal reactions. Attitude may affect tests of one particular kind, because of associations which they arouse. In some cases it may be that under the stress of emotion the individual is unable to adjust himself to novel situations, to show any planfulness or initiative, whereas tasks that require mere memory or which can be readily performed on the basis of long established reactions or habits, are unaffected by the stress under which the individual is laboring. Instances of this kind have been reported elsewhere at length.[1]

In all psychological examinations one must rule out the factor of *simulation* before accepting a negative result at its face value. Because of some special consideration, the individual may simulate general disability, or he may feign inability to perform some special kind of work, in accordance with some plan or purpose of his

[1] Bronner, Augusta F., "Attitude as it Affects Performance of Tests." *Psychological Review*, July, 1916.

own. We have known cases in institutions where the individual did not wish to be held in the schoolroom, preferring, possibly, other activities, and he therefore pretended to be unable to do the work demanded by the school teacher. On tests one sometimes finds an individual who shows very distinct dislike for some type of work, and who, because of his simulation of disability, might be considered an instance of specialized defect were one not careful in the analysis of results.

In distinguishing between general defect and normality accompanied by special defect, there are several points to be considered. Before concluding that an individual is a defective, that is, feeble-minded, there should be several kinds of evidence, each of which corroborates the other. Unfortunately, the practice of basing the diagnosis of feeble-mindedness merely on the results of Binet or other "measuring scales" is all too common. Sometimes grave errors are made, particularly when the subject is handicapped by either a lack of adequate knowledge of English or by a special defect for language. The proper emphasis on the social implications of feeble-mindedness is a help, but several other considerations should play a part.

From our long experience we are convinced that for the diagnosis of feeble-mindedness there should be given not only (a) the Binet tests, but also (b) a number of performance tests, to which should be added (c) the individual's reactions to ordinary or common-sense situations, and (d) the extent to which he has profited by educational opportunities. When these four types of tests are used, the final conclusions reached should be fair and valid, provided the tests have been made under favorable conditions. All of the disturbing factors above enumerated, of course, must be absent. If diagnosis is based on less evidence than is here set forth, there is always a possibility, among other things, that what is designated feeble-mindedness may, in reality, be only special defect.

To distinguish between the normal individual with special disability and the defective with special ability should not present a very difficult problem in the light of all that we have already said. When failure is confined to tests which involve some special mental process or processes, and all other types of tests are done well, it is more than likely that the individual is normal, but with some special defect. When, on the other hand, tests involving varied mental processes are performed poorly, with the exception of a group which depends upon some one mental process, it is more likely that the individual is a defective with some special ability. This ability or disability may involve language, memory, motor reactions, or any other mental activity. When the results on various tests do not correlate and a marked discrepancy is found, it becomes necessary to evaluate results in the light of all the considerations we have discussed.

It will readily be seen that the problem of mental diagnosis is exceedingly complex, not always easy of solution. In order that the verdict may be sane and fair and present a prognosis and recommendations that are practically valuable, there must be intensive study of each individual problem case. We may repeat that this necessitates psychological examination so complete and the use of tests so diversified that some knowledge may be obtained of the various aspects of mental life. But this psychological examination is not sufficient. There must be included, above all, the developmental history, which often illuminates the whole problem, the physical conditions at the time of examination, the educational opportunities which the individual has had, the social background, and perhaps the facts of heredity. It is the accuracy and the completeness of all these data which determine the value of the final diagnosis.

CHAPTER IV

SOME PRESENT EDUCATIONAL TENDENCIES

IT is of interest to review briefly the main trends of present-day tendencies in education, to discover, if we can, to what extent they are concerned with the problems of special ability and special defect. There is at present a great awakening in the educational world, an appreciation of the fact that in the past many principles have been accepted as true without an effort being made to establish them on scientific bases. Logical deductions were earlier the chief justification for procedure; then psychological laws became the criteria, but largely without any study of their applicability to specific situations, or of their truth and value under definite and varying conditions.

To-day the recognition of the fallacies to which this mode of thinking lead is becoming widespread. In consequence, questions are arising concerning the aims of education and the methods of attaining them. Experimentation is being undertaken in the hope of learning how desired goals may be best achieved. This spirit of inquiry is affecting all aspects of education — curricula, methods, schemes of school administration — and is leading to studies of applied psychology dealing with the separate mental processes, with laws of learning, and with means of measuring and evaluating actual school results.

In general, the main interests so far have centered about the formulation and application of general principles. It seems fair to state that the product of education has been considered more than the process, the group more than the individual. School researches, as a whole, have dealt very little with attempts at analysis of the underlying and conditioning factors of the learning process. They have stressed the measurement of results of educational practice, but not the reasons for success or failure. They have investigated school systems as a whole, but not the individuals who comprise the school systems.

While nearly all studies in experimental psychology prove the fact of individual differences, little effort has been made to show the practical correlations in adaptation of method and subject matter that must naturally follow in order to meet adequately the individual differences which exist. But since one salient characteristic of the mental life is individual differences, this certainly should affect the theory of education on the one hand and practical procedure on the other. The lack of experimentation in the field of individual needs is noteworthy; it is undoubtedly on account of this that the problems of individual special defect or of unusual ability have been largely disregarded.

Let us review briefly some specific examples illustrating the main trends of educational theory and practice, regarding them critically in relation to the problem of the individual.

The aim of education most frequently stressed at the present time is perhaps best expressed as the socialization of the individual. Though the evolution of this ideal cannot here be presented, nor the arguments in its behalf, nor the consequences to which it has led, it may be said that even so broad and alluring a principle has taken little account of the practical means for reaching each individual and socializing him. The fact that in order to attain this ideal for each individual the means must be varied, has been virtually disregarded. It has been implied, if not specifically stated, that the same scheme of education, the same studies and the same methods, are equally successful for all children. The schools founded on this philosophy and purporting to accomplish this end presumably hope to achieve it by adopting the same procedure for all. So splendid and inspiring a presentation as that made in Dewey's recent book [1] gives little heed to individual variations in abilities, at least as a fundamental aspect of human life that must form one of the chief principles in education. Nor do schools that stand most strongly for the embodiment of this view of education as a socializing process pay much more heed to individual adjustments than schools that are supposedly less progressive and liberal.

However widely such a general end as the socialization of the individual may be applicable, it requires adaptation of method to individual characteristics for its accomplishment. And herein lies one great weakness, it would seem, in present-day tendencies. Method is one aspect of education that has been much discussed; volumes have been written on both general method and special methods pertaining to the different school subjects, but until recently there has been little attempt to make method a rational outgrowth of psychological findings. Freeman's recent book [2] purports to show the application of psychological laws to problems of instruction, but little or no cognizance is taken of the relation to the mental make-up of the individual.

In some schools of education, studies are now being

[1] Dewey, John, "Democracy and Education", 1916.
[2] Freeman, Frank N., "The Psychology of the Common Branches", 1916.

carried on in an effort to establish the psychology of such studies as arithmetic, spelling, and reading, and other of the usual schoolroom activities. Here, as in study of the more elemental psychological processes, experimentation must gather the data and establish the general laws.

We need to know the psychological laws related to learning in the different school subjects, laws which apply to the majority and which will be effective with the greater portion of the school population. We are just beginning to realize the intricacy and complexity of the mental processes that are brought into play in ordinary school subjects popularly thought to be simple. But it should be added that even after such generalizations are reached, there will always remain the problem of the individual who presents special conditions. Individual differences will ever be extreme enough to make many exceptions to the general rule. Some children will always require special consideration and special adaptation of both subject matter and method. The ideal of teaching efficiently individuals with special defect or special ability can be realized only after we are able to analyze the situations they present and to direct practical efforts in accordance with established principles of learning the various subjects. Study of individuals and knowledge of method should have a reciprocal relationship, the development of each aiding the progress of the other.

After all, the practicability of an end, in education as elsewhere, and the value of the means used to attain the end can only be determined by the results achieved. The evaluation of accomplishment is a distinct feature of present activities in educational circles, much more so than at any period in the past. One evidence of this is seen in the number of surveys which so many cities have undertaken for the purpose of determining the efficiency of their school systems.

Another proof of the tendency to measure educational product is evidenced by the rapidity with which objective scales for measuring achievement in the various school subjects have been evolved. By means of these scales it is proposed to estimaté progress from time to time and to compare results obtained by the use of various methods in teaching. In scales, as in school surveys, it is product that is being studied and not process. Such methods of evaluation are a very practicable help since they obviate the use of subjective and hence very unreliable standards. But they throw no light whatsoever upon the reasons for success or failure, nor is much clue given in explanation of the advantage which one method or one system has over another. Measuring scales make it possible to compare an individual's ability with a norm for his age, or with the achievement of any other individual, and to gauge his own progress from time to time, but they do not touch upon the mental processes involved in any activity. They are concerned with complex achievements, not with the separate aspects of mental life, hence they are of little use in the study of problem cases.

The inadequacy of this type of investigation may be illustrated by discussing briefly the problems of retardation and elimination, both naturally related to our present subject. We may judge of their seriousness and practical import by the number of published studies dealing with these topics. Retardation has been discussed from the standpoint of its extent, both in terms of the percentage of the school population that is retarded and the number of years of retardation. Very little study has been made, however, of the causes of retardation or the characteristics of retarded individuals. It seems strange, indeed, that no one has endeavored to make any thorough analysis of this problem from the standpoint of causation, an analysis that would seem possible on the basis of intensive study of an unselected, representative group of retarded children. In studies of the elimination of children from school, the main concern has been to determine the percentage of those who withdraw at each school grade. Van Denburg's [1] more thorough study of the conditions affecting elimination in the public high schools of New York City covers the nationality and occupation of the parents, the educational and vocational careers of older brothers and sisters, the economic status of the family, the pupils' valuation of a high school education and the occupations in which they hoped to engage. But interesting as this study is and valuable as is the information it gives regarding the force of certain environmental and home conditions, it takes little account of the influence of one possibly very important factor, namely, lack of adjustment of the course of study to the interest and capacity of the individual student. Van Denburg recognizes this as one element, though he offers no data on the point. In the chapter entitled "New Courses and New Types of Schools", he says, "Among the many conclusions possible there seems at least one conclusion that we all must draw from this investigation taken as a whole, namely that an extremely large percentage of the population enters high school unwilling or unable to benefit properly by the instruction which is offered at present. . . . To permit the pupils to drag along in courses for which they have no aptitude and in which they are visibly receiving little benefit is equally unjust, particularly to the city which provides, at so great an expense, costly and capable instruction." It is evident that this is equally unjust to the pupils who are spending their time in schools whose function avowedly is to educate them. We are in great

[1] Van Denburg, J. K., "Causes of Elimination of Students in Public Secondary Schools of New York City", 1911.

need of duplication of this type of investigation in regard to elimination in the lower grades, particularly from the standpoint of the ability of the child as correlated with courses that are offered.

It is true the school has not been altogether unaware of this failure in the past to meet the needs of all children, and some few measures have been undertaken, both as regards administration and courses of study, to improve the situation. On the administrative side certain exceedingly interesting innovations are being tried in an effort to make the school a more flexible organization. The inauguration of pre-vocational schools, the organizing of the school into two six-year divisions instead of an eight-year grammar-school course followed by a four-year high-school course, the plan of one continuous twelve-year course — all these are examples of present-day attempts to improve school administration in order to reach the individual more effectively.

Related to this same problem of adjustment to meet individual ability and interest is the present-day tendency toward establishing more and more elective courses. There is no doubt that this newer feature of our schools is partly based upon the recognition of the principle that all children are not equally able to benefit by the same training. Granting the wisdom of this differentiation of courses, there still remains the question of the basis on which the selection is to be made. Is present selection of courses made in accordance with each individual's ability in the various fields, and upon whose judgment does the selection rest? Too frequently considerations that are not really valid enter into the decision. The child himself may be influenced by the choice of friends, or by the idea that one course is easier than another, or the parents may make the decision for him according to some preconceived notion of what constitutes an education. Too little consideration is given to the adaptability of the child for the courses that are offered, and his past successes and failures are frequently not regarded as essential in the choice.

Then, too, this liberal attitude is found only in high school or in the year or two preceding it. Probably the introduction of elective courses is not practicable in the lower grades, where the subject matter is of such a character that all children require it, but even there recognition of the principle of individual needs is wise, if only for the adaptation of methods of teaching in special cases.

Concerning courses of study there is at present much discussion, but very little in the way of definite conclusion. All of us are familiar with the fact that new subjects are being added to the curriculum, and that there is great difference of opinion in regard to the advisability of retaining many of them. On the one hand, we find those who believe that we still should continue the old type of education which stressed the three R's and included some subjects unrelated to practical life, but believed to be of disciplinary value. On the other hand, there are those who think that information and mental discipline apart from the activities of daily life do not accomplish the desired end. They say real education consists in developing power over the forces of social life, and that all selection of topics and methods should be worked out in accordance with the intrinsic social value of the content.

The whole problem is involved, and it is not intended to enter into the controversy except as it applies to individuals with special defects or with special abilities. In these cases school work must be adapted to the unusual conditions if the individual is to be educated. The typical school and vocational failures that are cited afford proof of the futility of any other point of view.

Consideration of vocational failures leads at once to

another group of problems now arousing much interest in the educational world, but as yet far from solved. The only one with which we are here concerned is the possibility of vocational guidance, particularly in its relation to educational diagnosis. Some of those who are closely identified with the movement for vocational guidance are skeptical of the help that psychological study of the individual offers. Our own feeling on the subject is that, while acknowledging the present limitations, one must recognize certain very definite possibilities of diagnosis even now, as well as the considerable hope for future development in this field. In general, it should be said that our knowledge of the mental processes required in various industries is very scanty and uncertain; until this knowledge is increased one cannot be sure of the correlations that exist between what is tested and industrial efficiency. Certainly, at the present time, subtle distinctions and definite statements concerning correlations can rarely be made. One cannot be sure that laboratory results would obtain if experimentation were made under the conditions of the workshop, where a number of other factors enter into the situation.[1]

Nevertheless, within wide limits, advice in regard to vocations may be safely made on the basis of results of psychological examinations. No one doubts for an instant that special disabilities preclude the possibility of success in certain fields of industrial endeavor. The case-histories given later illustrate the fact that some grave errors might be avoided in the placing of boys and girls in the industrial world.

Though one trend of the present is the assumption by

[1] A recent book by H. L. Hollingworth ("Vocational Psychology", 1916) summarizes the present possibilities in this field, indicates the general methods that have thus far been employed in efforts toward vocational testing, and enumerates some of the tests that are helpful for this purpose.

the school of a certain amount of responsibility for obtaining positions for boys and girls, yet little cognizance is taken of qualities and abilities or disabilities that later become important factors in vocational success. The irrationality of our present scheme, which takes no account even of such characterizations of prospective employés as teachers could give on the basis of their knowledge of children, quite apart from psychological study, leads to great waste. One great hope for future better vocational adjustment is through the application of what can be learned during school life by teachers and clinical psychologists of special fitness for different industrial occupations.

Interpretation of all the movements we have briefly reviewed from the point of view of their purpose, strengthens our thesis that intensive observation of individuals is complementary to investigation of whole groups. Through individual diagnosis such as we have outlined in the previous chapters, much may be learned that will have direct application to changes in subjects to be taught and methods to be used, at least in problem cases, as well as in applying to vocational guidance what may be learned through studying the facts of individual differences.

CHAPTER V

SPECIAL DEFECTS IN NUMBER WORK

NOT long ago the statement was made by Suzzallo [1] that "attempts to inquire into the special psychology of the arithmetical processes through experimentation and control have not been numerous or influential on current practice." Indeed, there is comparatively little literature bearing upon any questions of experimental pedagogy, Meumann's recent book being the first attempt at any thorough or complete presentation of the problems [2] or of solutions in so far as they are based on either analysis or experimentation. A few thinkers have endeavored to determine the psychological processes that underlie number work, but little has been written on the subject, compared with the volumes which discuss methods and devices from a logical rather than from a psychological standpoint.

As long ago as 1897, McLennan and Dewey,[3] writing on the psychology of number, devoted considerable discussion to the mental processes involved. The point of view presented is that number is a rational concept, not a sense fact, that it has its basis in concrete experience, and that it involves, in the main, the psychological processes of discrimination and generalization, under

[1] Suzzallo, Henry, "The Teaching of Primary Arithmetic ", 1912.
[2] Meumann, Ernst, "Vorlesungen zur Einführung in die Experimentelle Pädagogik ", 1914.
[3] McLennan and Dewey, "Psychology of Number ", 1897.

50

which latter head are included abstraction and the power of grouping. Discrimination leads the child to a recognition of objects as units; from undefined wholes he advances to a concept of separate parts. On the other hand, he learns by his own activity to combine parts into definite wholes; he sees separate objects as a group or unity. Thus, it is by the power of abstraction that he comes to neglect all characteristic qualities of an object other than its number. When he gathers like units into a whole he has advanced to the second step in generalization, namely, to grouping. Hence, these authors conclude that the concept of number cannot be taught by the mere presentation of things, but only by such a presentation as will stimulate discrimination and abstraction, as previously explained. Or, to express the idea somewhat differently, we might say that these writers emphasize the fact that there may be clear percepts of things quite unaccompanied by definite numerical concepts. The development of these numerical concepts requires the child to compare and relate, to discriminate and generalize.

Lanner, in his article, "Wie Lernt das Kind Zählen?"[1] discusses the development which takes place from the stage at which the child uses numerical terms as names without numerical significance, and the stage at which numerical terms express a real concept of number. The realization of this difference is shown by Binet when he cautions against accepting the child's ability to say numerals serially as equivalent to the power to count the number of objects in a group.

The most thorough discussion of the whole problem is to be found in Meumann's chapter on the subject. He, too, feels that there has been as yet no adequate analysis

[1] Lanner, A., "Wie Lernt das Kind Zählen?" *Zeitschrift für Philosophie und Pädagogik*, 1903.

of the mental processes involved and that the study of the development of number concept, frequently reached before school age, has hardly been undertaken. He states that Pestalozzi was the first to formulate any underlying principles and his only contribution concerns basing the teaching of arithmetic on perception of objects, after which there should follow a study of the grouping of objects and of their relationship to each other.

Meumann agrees in general with this point of view, but discusses much more in detail the psychology of the subject. He states that the concept of number develops late, that it rests upon a basis of counting objects, and from this experience with the concrete there gradually grows an understanding of abstract number relations, while counting itself becomes purely mechanical. The stage of development of number concept with which children enter school varies greatly and depends largely upon environmental opportunities. Eckhardt's experiments [1] have shown this, and in measuring scales for intelligence, such as the Binet-Simon and the Terman-Childs, tests involving numbers are placed relatively late. This late development is to be accounted for by the fact that some of the higher mental processes, such as abstraction, analysis, and comprehension, are required. It is only by abstracting from the concrete background that the idea of number, as such, is evolved. The child analyzes his own experience and ultimately reaches a comprehension of the function of number.

But performance in elementary arithmetic involves several other main factors. The mechanical manipulation of the fundamental steps requires memory for number and the formation of arbitrary associations. It is upon these two mental processes that both accuracy and speed

[1] Eckhardt, K., "Beobachtungen über das Zahlenverständnis der Schulrekruten." *Zeitschrift für experimentelle Pädagogik*, 8, 1909.

are based; by means of memory definite habits of reaction are established so that arithmetic can be performed without thinking over the various steps in a problem.

Nowhere have I found a summary such as the following which combines the partial analyses of various writers. (1) The concept of number is built up through actual experience in handling objects. (2) On the basis of this active experience there is evolved a comprehension of the function of number on the one hand, and of numerical relationships on the other. (3) To succeed in the process of evolving a complete concept of number, the child needs to analyze and compare, to discriminate, and finally to abstract; that is, there must be ultimately a transition from concrete to abstract. (4) Memory processes are implicated and particularly essential in the mechanical aspects of number manipulation. (5) Arbitrary association is an element in the learning process.

Concerning the rôle played by other subsidiary mental functions, there is considerable disagreement, for example, regarding the relationship of the various types of imagery. Eckhardt [1] endeavored to find by experimentation what significance visual elements have for memory for numbers and for the performance of the fundamental operations. His conclusion is that children who visualize well use this type of imagery in their arithmetic work, and that it is a great help to them. He believes that these children are superior both in memory for number and readiness in counting. He urges that all types be trained to use visual imagery in number work, since he believes it to be such a great advantage. Children who predominantly visualize may be somewhat slower, but they are far more accurate, according to his findings.

[1] Eckhardt, K., "Visuelle Erinnerungsbilder beim Rechnen." *Zeitschrift für experimentelle Pädagogik*, 5, 1907.

Lobsien,[1] on the other hand, offers proof of the opposite. He found in his experimentation a fairly high correlation between auditory memory and facility in both written and oral arithmetic, whereas there was an inverse relationship between visual memory and written and oral arithmetic. It is but fair to add that there has been criticism of both these studies, and the problem at present remains largely unsettled.

It can readily be seen that in certain aspects arithmetic depends upon other functions. Thus, in the solving of arithmetical problems, reason often is involved. The place of reasoning in the teaching of mechanical features of arithmetic leads us to a further problem. It is evident that in learning the fundamental processes — addition, subtraction, multiplication, and division — memory alone may be relied on very largely, and no doubt very many children learn number combinations and their manipulations on the basis of sheer rote memory. They are rarely taught, nor do they perhaps need to know the rationalities, for example of the decimal system. They know that in addition of two-place numbers, one adds the digits of the right-hand column and puts in the answer the unit number of the total and "carries" the remainder to be added to the integers of the left-hand column. The "borrowing" of a number in subtraction is learned without any explanation of the logic back of the performance. In most instances the child does as he is told to do by the teacher, and through practice establishes definite habits of reaction in given situations.

Suzzallo has discussed at length the principles upon which to decide whether habituation or rationalization shall be stressed. The point to be here added is that,

---

[1] Lobsien, M., "Korrelation zwischen Zahlengedächtnis und Rechenwertung." *Zeitschrift für Pädagogische Psychologie*, 1911.

valid as his generalizations may be for the majority of children, there are instances where specialized defects of one kind or another may require that other than ordinary procedures be adopted.

If now, in our study of individual problem cases, we find a child who is greatly retarded in number work, who seems to be incapable of normal advancement in this subject, it becomes necessary to make such an intensive investigation by means of psychological tests that we shall be able, if possible, to determine wherein the difficulty lies. If we know the psychological processes involved in the learning of arithmetic, we ought to test these various mental functions in the individual in order to find which are normal and which are not. Since memory for number and the ability to form arbitrary associations are elements in the learning of number work on the mechanical side, we must find whether these processes function normally in each individual case. Furthermore, the more fundamental problems must likewise be answered, namely, whether the child has any concept of number and, if so, whether he has been able to form those abstractions which are necessary in the performance of the usual school tasks. Perhaps he is able to solve problems when using concrete material and yet not able to perform correctly abstract work.

On the other hand, it may be that the methods which are ordinarily successful fail. It is quite conceivable that whereas habituation may be usually quite adequate, rationalization should be substituted in certain specific cases where memory powers are particularly faulty. Herein may lie the explanation of a fact pointed out by Judd,[1] that in the same school system some children have been found who succeed better on work in

¹ Judd, C. H., "Survey of Cleveland Schools." "The Cleveland Foundation", 1916.

arithmetic of the advanced grades than previously in the lower grades. That this cannot be due to general poor teaching is proven, since it is not a feature of the class as a whole, but only of certain individuals.

Before concluding that failure in any individual is due to special defect, it is necessary, of course, to be careful not to confuse this with the effects of poor teaching. Sometimes the teaching has been such that certain fundamental principles have not been thoroughly established, and the child may do much of the work correctly, but have trouble with some one step in the processes. He may be able to do the higher work and yet fail in some of the easier steps. For example, a child may be quite accurate in multiplication and addition and yet not perform subtraction correctly; or he may never have been taught the correct use of the zero, so that wherever this is involved, errors are made. Of course, this is a matter of poor and inadequate teaching rather than any difficulty with the child.

A number of cases are here presented, in all of which there is one common feature, namely, the individual proves himself normal, except for special disability in number work. The question is whether the mental processes as studied by psychological tests can be analyzed in order to explain the defect that is found.

Case 7. The following illustration of inability in number work probably rests on a basis of an exceeding defect in auditory memory for numbers, uncompensated for by training suited to special characteristics.

Willard Z., 15½ years old, was studied on several occasions and at considerable length. It was found that he did many things very well, including tests of such difficulty as to prove that the boy was, in general, quite capable. In marked contradistinction to results on other tests and other school subjects, we found that he was an absolute failure in the handling of numbers. He failed on each of the four fundamental processes; he could not add four three-place numbers correctly, nor could he subtract, multiply, or divide. Although he had learned the multiplication table by rote, yet when he tried to use it he became confused, made many errors, and did not succeed in getting a correct answer in any of a number of examples given.

Even more amazing was the fact that the boy could not make the simplest change, in spite of the fact that he had been employed for months and consequently had handled money. His mother told us that she could not send him to the store to make any purchases because he did not know if the correct change were given him. We found that he could not tell how much money would be left from half a dollar if thirty-six cents were spent, nor the change left from a dollar after eighty-seven cents worth of goods had been purchased, When the money was before him he could not make change; indeed, in this last problem, he told us that twenty-seven cents would be left, but even this he could not actually count out. He made change correctly only when handling nickels or multiples thereof. In an effort to perform very simple problems orally he became altogether confused. This was true whether reasoning was involved or not. He tried very hard, without success, to find the cost of two thirds of a dozen oranges when a dozen cost twenty-four cents; he could not tell the cost of eight articles if five cost a quarter. He was no more successful in giving the answer to the following, How much is $(7 + 8 + 3) \times 2$? He added change totaling $1.25 correctly, but even here he did this by counting by nickels and dimes.

Construction tests were done extremely well, by a thoroughly rational method and with a quick perception of relationships. Tests for mental representation and analysis, while more difficult for him, were accomplished successfully. He showed on tests very good apperceptions, normal control of verbal associations, and normal ability to form new associations. He followed directions well. Judged by the Binet scale he was normal in ability. None of the tests for separate mental functions thus far enumerated occasioned him any difficulty; they were performed rapidly and readily.

When memory powers were studied, remarkable findings were obtained. Rote visual memory was normal. He accurately reproduced drawings shown him, but it was a different story when auditory powers were tested. To our great amazement we found that the boy could remember only four numerals, and although tested on different occasions and given a great many trials, he never succeeded in repeating five numerals presented auditorily. He did, on the other hand, repeat seven numerals given visually. As for logical material, he gave fifteen out of twenty items when he himself read a passage, and eight out of twelve items when the passage was read to him — results that are better in comparison than those for rote memory. Thus we see that while visual memory tests presented no peculiarity, the achievement on the rote auditory tests was worse than that expected of a normal eight-year-old child. The auditory memory powers of many low grade feeble-minded are far better than those of this otherwise capable boy.

He read fluently and with good expression. He was able to give a correct reproduction of the main ideas contained in the passage read, except that here his inability to remember numbers was again evident. He reproduced correctly the substance of a "help wanted" advertisement, except for the numbers given. He could not remember the number of the office building nor the number of the room where the applicant should apply. He wrote a legible hand and spelled correctly all the words given him in a fairly difficult dictation.

The boy was quite conscious of his own defect in number work and after leaving regular school and beginning to work he had attended night school hoping to gain there some knowledge of arithmetic. He had gone for three weeks and then stopped, quite discouraged. He realized that all his school career had been hampered by his difficulty, and, indeed, he had only reached fourth grade in spite of his very evident capacity for acquiring knowledge of many kinds.

Except in the light of his successes and failures on psychological tests, it would be difficult to explain his inability to learn arithmetic by ordinary methods. One could only have concluded without tests that he has a very specialized defect, but there could be no understanding of the basis for it. The explanation is evident when his exceedingly poor auditory memory for numbers is discovered. One may ask whether the boy had any concept of number. Certain it is he has had opportunity for acquiring this if only through his experience while working. As for powers of discrimination and abstraction, which are involved in the transition from experience with the concrete to facility with abstract number combinations, no defect for these is found on tests. If they are at fault and are factors in his inability to perform arithmetic work, they are at least specialized and true only in this one field.

It is impossible to state definitely whether any amount of training would have overcome this innate lack; it is certain that now, at his age, it would still be unprofitable to endeavor to teach him by the usual methods, which have already proved ineffectual in his case, since his training had been extended over more than eight years.

The only recommendation one could make in such a case is that the boy should be taught by a method adapted to his mental peculiarities. Since he has such poor auditory memory, one could hardly rely upon mere rote auditory training and drill. It would seem wiser to use his good powers of reasoning and visualization and to teach by a method which might be for the majority uneconomical and clumsy.

The social implications of the boy's defect are difficult to measure. Willard had been in court several times because of sex delinquencies. His mind seemed fairly obsessed by bad sex ideas; he had written several obscene letters. His actions can be accounted for partly, at least, on the basis of sex knowledge learned at a school to which he had been sent about two years previously. Furthermore, the boy was in the midst of adolescence and premature in sexual development. It cannot be definitely stated that his lack of ability for certain mental tasks had any direct relation to his misconduct, but, on the other hand, it is a fair assumption that had his school progress been altogether normal, he might have developed good mental interests which would have been sufficiently strong to prevent the growth of delinquent tendencies which he showed. There is a possibility that the low grade he reached in school and the discouragements resulting therefrom were factors in his career.

We learned that the heredity in the case was not good. The father had been alcoholic and abusive, had deserted his family when Willard was three years old. The mother had later obtained a divorce. She herself appeared to be a good and normal woman. The developmental history was negative, and environmental conditions had been fairly satisfactory, except during the time that the boy attended the school mentioned above.

His physical development was normal except for sex

prematurity. He had extremely defective vision, partly corrected by glasses. It was claimed that his vision had been affected by an accident which occurred a couple of years previously, when he had been hit in the temple by a rock. There was a small scar over one eye and some bone involvement. All other findings on the physical side were negative.

Case 8. Next is given an illustration of defect for number work where there is not merely poor auditory memory, but this is combined with poor powers of forming associations with symbolic material.

Alfred T., 16½ years old, was found on mental tests to be quite irregular in his abilities and disabilities. In spite of good educational advantages, the results on school work were not at all satisfactory, and particularly was this true in the field of arithmetic. He read only fairly well, making errors on small words, showing not so much a disability as a lack of facility; that is, he was quite inaccurate and careless in his reading, his failures being often on simple words, whereas difficult portions of the passage were read correctly. He wrote a childish hand and made some errors in writing from dictation. However, more striking was the fact that, although he had been attending business college for the purpose of becoming a bookkeeper, he was unable to add correctly five three-place numerals. He worked at this very painstakingly and slowly. He had not the slightest conception of the solution of problems such as interest, though at the time he was receiving practice in this at school. He very frankly said that he could not remember the bookkeeping work.

He did tests with concrete material remarkably well, attaining excellent records. He showed not only quick perception, but good reasoning powers in such work, and proved to have extremely good psychomotor control as well. On the other hand, his work with abstract material was not nearly as well done. He made a very poor record on the so-called learning test, where the association of arbitrary symbols is involved. This test, readily performed correctly by bright eight-year-old children, was most difficult for him, and the result was far below normal. His control of verbal associations was likewise not good; he made a very poor record on the opposites test. Concerning powers of analysis, the results were rather irregular, the test-findings differed one from the other. Memory powers seemed to be unequal, visual memory being better than auditory. In reproducing a passage presented visually, he omitted only three out of twenty items, whereas in the passage presented by auditory means he omitted four out of twelve items and altered other details.

His social reactions corroborated the test results which indicated his special abilities and defects. Alfred was the youngest of four children, the other three of whom had been through school and business college and had been successful in office work. The parents were intelligent people of foreign birth, and the family was distinctly on the upgrade. They were proud of the success of their other children and anxious to give this boy an equally good education, which they conceived would best be acquired through training in a business college.

Alfred had attended public school for eight years, where he reached the seventh grade; then, at fourteen, he wished to go to work. He had been employed at times, but had attended night school for seven months, after which he was sent by his parents to a business college in order to prepare him for bookkeeping. Just before leaving the public school he had been truant for three weeks. This was the beginning of his misconduct. Later, while attending business college, he ran away from home and repeated this frequently thereafter, being gone as long as a month at a time. He was brought into court on two occasions because of this and once because he stole a revolver, the only known instance of theft on his part.

During his absences from home he made his own way, frequently by selling papers and once by working at a livery stable. His employment record was good; he had worked at one place for seven months, but had given up this job because it was too hard for him. It was after this that the family sent him to the business college in hopes of "making a gentleman of him, the same as the others in the family."

He was a big, strong boy, well developed and well nourished. His tonsils were greatly enlarged, and there was a total occlusion of one side of the nose from deflected septum. Vision was somewhat defective in one eye, but almost normal in the other. There was a constant fine tremor of outstretched hands and biting of the finger nails, indicating some nervousness.

His delinquencies, that is, his truancy and running away, were due, no doubt, to several causes. They had begun while his mother was away on a visit to her parents, and oversight at home consequently was slackened. He had associated with bad companions who had led him to run away, but it is interesting to note that the first escapade of this sort was during the time he was attending the business college. Then, too, there was probably some irritation because of his physical troubles, particularly his defective vision, which may have interfered with his school work. Also, he was an unstable adolescent.

Nevertheless, there is not the slightest doubt that one important factor in explaining the boy's misconduct was the unsuitable vocation for which he was being trained.

He had not the slightest interest in bookkeeping and he was not fitted for the work. His people, well intentioned, did not appreciate the true situation; they only felt that they were offering the best means to success such as his brothers and sisters had achieved. That the boy liked best driving and working with horses and that he had been able to take care of himself by working in these ways when he was away from home, did not mean anything to them, whereas it can readily be seen that even the association with bad companions might have been explained through the lack of interest the boy felt in his forced occupation. Had he been busily engaged in pursuits which held his interest he might never have sought such companionship or have been so ready to follow suggestions made.

The proof that these points were vital matters for his whole career is shown by the fact that, acting upon advice given in the light of psychological findings, the boy was placed at farm work, and now, five years after he was first seen, we hear that he is still in the country and doing very well. He has worked satisfactorily, is earning good wages, was long ago released from court supervision, and is apparently happy with his station in life. His family have recognized the facts in the case and are themselves quite reconciled to his career as a farmer.

Certainly the study of this boy was well worth while, and the practical results based upon the findings of this study are conclusive evidence of the social importance involved in the recognition of special abilities and disabilities. The educational applications cannot be so definitely stated, because when seen the boy was too old to make it practicable to give him any individual training. Had he been considerably younger one might have suggested definite methods whereby he would have improved, perhaps, in certain directions. Knowing that he was particularly poor in dealing with abstractions and likewise somewhat below par in auditory memory powers, arithmetic might have been approached from the concrete aspects and with emphasis on visual memory as a means of control.

In any case, the school had not met his needs adequately. Had the special defect been so excessive that the boy could not be taught arithmetic even by adapted methods, the school should have been aware of the necessity for so guiding the boy vocationally that he might have avoided sure failure. The school authorities should have been able to give to the parents the advice which was offered at the time of our study.

Case 9. In this case is illustrated the fact that with normal ability to form arbitrary associations and with no defect in memory for numbers, there still may be failure in arithmetic because the concept of number is lacking.

Mary L., 11 years old, appeared at first as extremely bright. She was such an alert, active girl, she talked so well and interestingly about many things, that she made a most favorable impression. On a wide range of tests for determining mental ability Mary did very well. She did construction tests in a rational manner; she showed good apperceptive ability; she had no difficulty in associating arbitrary symbols and learned them with ease. On the Binet scale she graded to age, but even more interesting was the fact that on the common-sense tests included in that scale she did exceedingly well. She showed much shrewdness and good judgment for a girl of her age; her sense of humor was keen, she very quickly perceived the absurd situations in the so-called incongruities test; her answers were always relevant and well expressed. Her memory powers for rote material were just about normal for her age, neither exceptionally good nor exceptionally poor. She had much difficulty with tests involving mental representation when the task was at all difficult.

In regard to her school work, she had learned to read fluently; she wrote a fairly good hand and had no difficulty whatever with spelling. Her school retardation — for she was only in the second grade — might have been due, in part, to early poor opportunities, as we shall see later, but her exceeding defect in number work would be enough to account for it. She had received private instruction during the vacation. In spite of this, now, when eleven years old, she could do none of the fundamental processes except addition, and even this was done very slowly. She could not succeed with so simple a sum as subtracting eighteen from twenty-five; it made no difference whether this was given her orally, as a written problem, or with actual money. She said that "taking seven from seven leaves seven." It was evident that the common sense which she used in other situations had never been called into play in number work, otherwise she would surely not have made so stupid a remark. While she had learned a few of the number combinations orally, she very readily became confused. From the comments which she frequently made, it was apparent that numbers and words relating to them were meaningless to her.

Our examination of this little girl showed that she had not the slightest concept of number. She was utterly unable to master the work of her class, because she had not the ability to grasp what was being done. Whether she could have made normal progress had the concept of number been developed first through dealing with number relationships in concrete material, we have no way of knowing, but we feel sure that without this, the girl would become more and more confused by ordinary classroom procedure in this subject. It may be that this lack of concept of number was due somewhat to poor powers of mental representation, for no doubt this concept is developed through mentally representing to oneself relationships which constitute number. But Mary's native common sense and good general intelligence make it very probable that with individual help of the right kind she could be given the proper start and that her progress thereafter would be rapid.

When we become acquainted with this little girl she had been adopted by some kindly people who had taken her from her own poor home, and we were never able to obtain a reliable account of either heredity or early environmental conditions. We know that when quite young she lived for a time in an institution. It may be that early she had poor educational opportunities, but for nearly two years, at least, she has had exceedingly good home conditions and splendid chances for education. Physically she was in excellent condition, except for slight strabismus corrected by glasses. She was strong and well developed.

Mary was easily able to do much higher work in other school studies and in consequence she was wasting much of her time in school. The feeling of incompetence and discouragement which would naturally be aroused in her through failure and by being thrown with children so much younger than herself was likely to be most injurious. The injustice of the situation is manifest.

Case 10. This case illustrates the point that if the concept of number is not developed early, the failure in arithmetic continues in spite of ordinary drill and training for a number of years.

John T., 14 years and 10 months of age, was brought for examination because of his lack of progress in school. The mental examination soon showed that the source of the trouble lay in a defect for number work. How to explain this defect was a more difficult matter. He could not add four three-place numbers; he could not subtract, multiply, or divide, nor could he answer the simplest problems given him orally. He said that eight apples and five apples together made fifteen. He knew the date and his age, but could not tell the year in which he was born. With a square box in his hand, after he was told one side was two inches long, he could not tell the total number of inches on the four sides. With actual money before him he could not make change. He failed to add simple amounts correctly; he knew that two dimes made twenty cents and two nickels ten cents, but when pennies were added to this his answers were ludicrously incorrect. Simple problems involving reason were beyond him, although his reasoning powers, as shown on other tests, were very good.

There was a great discrepancy between results on tests for arithmetical ability and all other performances. Problems with concrete material were solved very well indeed. There was quick perception of the relationships involved, and rational methods were used in the solutions. General powers of apperception were quite normal, and this was true of memory processes and powers of representation. The rote memory tests were done very well; there was no difficulty with memory for numbers; the boy could restate correctly problems which he could not answer. He had learned in rote fashion the multiplication tables. His general intelligence, as gauged by Binet tests, was normal for his age. Reading, writing, and spelling were all performed satisfactorily.

That the concept of number was so entirely lacking could be explained, no doubt, only on the basis of some innate defect. The mother told us that she herself had attempted to teach the boy numbers when he was quite small, even before he was sent to school, but in regard to arithmetic "it was as if he were color blind." She could not send him to make purchases because he never knew if he had the correct change. His teachers had recognized his inability in this school subject, but no one had been able to help him. Just what methods of help had been employed we did not learn.

From the very intelligent, reliable mother we were able to obtain a thorough account of heredity and developmental history, both of which were altogether negative. The physical examination, made with care, revealed no sensory or other troubles.

It was quite apparent that the boy's disability had been a great influence in his school career. He had only reached the fifth grade when we saw him, whereas a sister, who began school at the same time as he, was already in the high school. Very fortunately, the boy was not sensitive in regard to his difficulty and his school retardation, and there was no complaint in regard to his behavior, except that he was exceedingly troublesome in the classroom. Just recently he had become a truant. Considering his handicap and that he was frequently forced to repeat his grade and was, in consequence, thrown constantly with younger children, it was surprising that he had not become more of a problem from the standpoint of his conduct.

Case 11. Sometimes, as in the following case, the difficulty is not easy to explain, for we may find almost all of the psychological processes which underlie number work quite normal. Here memory for numbers and powers of arbitrary association are not defective, nor is there any lack of ability to form mental representations. On the other hand, the step from the concrete to the abstract seems never to have been well established.

Henry M., 11 years old, was found exceedingly incapable in number work. In spite of his exceptionally good educational opportunities — good at least as ordinarily judged — he was unable to perform correctly any of the fundamental processes; he could not add, subtract, multiply, or divide. He had only slight knowledge of the multiplication tables, and he could not carry out the process of multiplication in even fairly simple problems. He failed to solve such easy oral examples as, if six cost twenty-four cents what will eight cost? It was quite evident that the boy had gained practically nothing from all his school training in number work. Other school subjects were done satisfactorily; he wrote a rapid, legible hand, misspelling words only occasionally. He read fluently and intelligently, and his reading had covered a wide range for a boy of his years.

We found he solved performance tests readily, making a remarkably good record both for speed and for accuracy. His records on construction tests are among the best ever made in our laboratory, even on those adapted for subjects much older than he. They prove that the boy has unusually good ability in the perception of relationships of form, in reasoning with concrete material, and in following directions with actual material when several steps are required. Nor was any difficulty shown on the so-called learning test, where the associations of arbitrary symbols were formed with ease. Memory power for both rote and logical material was normal for his age. Apperception was quite normal, and tests for analysis and mental representation were likewise well done. Indeed, there was conclusive proof that the boy had very good native ability in many directions.

Since this boy was first seen some four years ago, we have had corroboration of his abilities and disabilities through frequent school reports. In several schools which he has attended his records in industrial work have been exceptionally good, the grade in one school having been 100. In arithmetic his standing has been consistently low. The last report stated that his mathematical sense is far below par, although he has been able to master a few of the mechanics of arithmetic. In informational subjects the boy has always shown a keen interest, and his knowledge of geography, history, and literature is beyond his school grade.

The results of our mental tests led us to believe that the explanation of his extreme incapacity for handling numbers rests upon poor powers of dealing with arithmetical abstractions. Certainly, in concrete fields this boy shows extremely good ability. That his memory powers are normal is indicated not only by the psychological tests for these mental processes, but likewise by the fact that he has been able to acquire such a good fund of information. On the other hand, numerical relationships which involve powers of abstraction and appreciation of relationships of a very abstract nature, are altogether wanting. Although the defect is surprising, considering the boy's other innate abilities, the fact that it exists is obvious enough. We can only conclude that there is a special defect which makes it difficult for him to develop a concept of number.

That this particular disability has been of great significance in his school career and has led to much irritation throughout his entire school life, goes without saying. The boy had been lowered repeatedly in his school grade and had come to regard himself as a school failure. After the case was studied it still remained practically impossible to obtain the training suited to his needs. In the private schools to which he has been subsequently sent no teacher evidently has appreciated the problem or understood the psychological aspects of the situation.

No special adaptation of method, such as is really required, has ever been attempted. In spite of the fact that this boy has attended school where industrial courses are given, we doubt whether the work in arithmetic has actually been based upon these courses. In consequence, the step from the concrete to the abstract has never been bridged, and the understanding of number relationships in the light of their use in solving real problems has never been evolved.

In this particular instance no other explanation of school retardation was found. The boy was in excellent physical condition, the parents coöperated with the school and evinced in every possible way their desire for the boy to advance normally.

To show that an ordinary amount of testing, such as is frequently given merely to differentiate mental normality from feeble-mindedness, is inadequate to determine the underlying processes upon which arithmetical defect rests, the following cases are offered. In both, the problems as presented to us were not educational or even vocational.

Case 12.   Lillian M., 15 years old, showed very good ability in many things, and yet she was utterly unable to solve very simple problems in arithmetic. In all motor tests given her she made records that were practically as good as is obtainable. She did well on tests which required analysis and mental representation. She showed good powers of mental control and normal apperceptions. In school work her record was normal, except for arithmetic. She could add correctly, though this was done slowly, but all other number work was a failure. She made errors in subtraction, could not multiply or do simple examples in long division. In her case it seemed clear that the girl had been promoted in school in spite of her inability to do the arithmetic work of her grades, but she was quite retarded, having only completed the fifth grade when she withdrew at fourteen years.

In this case it was impracticable for the girl to receive any further training, and since her problem required only a verdict regarding normality, no other tests were given. From such findings we get little aid in discovering the basis for failure to master arithmetic. We are quite sure that there is a defect, but which of the underlying processes might explain it we do not know.

Case 13. Arthur L., 17 years old, showed on mental examination his inability to grasp number work. At seventeen he was only in the sixth grade, no doubt because of his special defect for numbers, for he was able to do other types of school work satisfactorily. Writing and spelling were done well, and he read a fairly difficult passage fluently, giving an accurate reproduction of the contents. That he was normal except in arithmetic was shown by the fact that he passed the 12-year Binet tests readily and showed normal powers of analysis and representation, normal powers in dealing with concrete material, and normal control of verbal associations.

In arithmetic, he failed in long division, making errors in multiplication and in subtraction; indeed, he showed no comprehension of any of the principles involved in number work. Even worse were the results on oral problems. He could not subtract $1.57 from $2.00, nor solve so simple a problem as the following: At thirty-six cents a dozen how much would five oranges cost? In the test for continuous subtraction he made many errors.

The point to be here emphasized is that routine and hurried testing, such as is frequently the custom even in connection with school laboratories, is insufficient for a rational understanding of these problem cases. Binet tests reveal nothing helpful in regard to the special defect, often not even indicating that it exists. To make the individual adjustments, which alone meet the situation adequately, much more intensive study is required, as indicated in the earlier cases cited.

CHAPTER VI

SPECIAL DEFECTS IN LANGUAGE ABILITY

FROM a practical standpoint it is found that the different aspects of language ability do not present a psychological unity. We know that defects in one or several aspects may exist without involving other phases. As a simple illustration of this, may be mentioned the fact that we frequently have studied individuals who have great difficulty in mastering reading, but who, nevertheless, speak well and seem to have no difficulty in the use of language as a medium of self-expression. This anomaly is very clearly shown in cases of feeble-minded verbalists, who, while unable to learn to read one language even fairly well, are able to converse in several. Then, too, we have known some who, while able to read quite well, have much difficulty in clear expression of their own ideas and little feeling for good use of language. Then there are those who are able to read fluently, but who cannot reproduce the ideas contained in the passage read. If all this is true, there must be distinct differences in the mental processes underlying language in its various aspects.

In discussing the topic of language, its teaching and the psychological principles involved, Meumann maintains that the whole field, from reading to the learning of foreign languages, is a unit psychologically considered, and that it must therefore be regarded as such pedagogically.   He includes the teaching of language, both native and foreign; reading, the interpretation of symbols; writing, the expression of ideas through the written word; and even drawing as a graphic representation of thought. Now, it seems clear to us that if these form a unity, there must be psychological processes common to all of them. Unfortunately, in spite of lengthy discussion of these different phases of language ability, Meumann does not tell us anywhere what the common elements actually are. In our own presentation of defects in language ability, we find the necessity for treating the various problems separately.

READING

In regard to the psychology of reading, it may be noted that much experimental work has been done on the part played by the eye, that is, on the physical aspects of the process.   Many experimenters have investigated the question of eye movements and the economics of perception.   It has been shown that the eye in its passage along a line pauses a number of times, and that it is during the pauses that we perceive the words.   The length of these pauses and the number of them to a line are influences in the rate of reading.   The formation of motor habits, the speed of reading in relation to length of line and size of print, the ease of grasping special words which can readily be grouped, as compared with those which cannot be so combined, have all been subjected to experimentation. Cattell [1], Erdmann and Dodge [2], Messmer [3], Dearborn [4],

[1] Cattell, J. McK., "Über die Zeit der Erkennung und Benennung von Schriftzeichen, Bildern und Farben."   "Wundt's Philosophische Studien", II, 1885, and III, 1886.

[2] Erdmann and Dodge, "Psychologische Untersuchungen über das Lesen", 1898.

[3] Messmer, O., "Zur Psychologie des Lesens bei Kindern und Erwachsenen", 1904.

[4] Dearborn, W. F., "The Psychology of Reading."   "Archives of Philosophy, Psychology and Scientific Methods", Vol. IV, 1906.

Hamilton [1], Huey [2], and others, have all made contributions in this field.

Much less, however, has been done to analyze the mental processes which are concerned in reading. Able though Huey's work is from certain standpoints, yet he hardly discusses the essential psychological phases of reading, and all his pedagogical advice is based upon what might be called the physiology of reading. Meumann, however, presents in some detail other factors. He mentions the problems of the visual apparatus on the one hand, and the ideational aspects on the other. He says words and the mental content which they represent are presented through sensory symbols, which must be seen and interpreted by the reader. There must be a recognition of letters and the association of them with sounds, after which combinations of letters become associated with combinations of sound, until whole words and phrases are recognized. These, in turn, are associated with meanings. Thus reading represents a complex activity based upon both analytical and synthetic processes. There are involved : perception and interpretation of symbols, memory — both recognition and recall of immediately preceding ideas, comprehension, motor processes, emotion, and complex associations.

There are a number of other questions that have a bearing on this general subject. One of these, the relationship of inner speech to ease and speed of reading, has been investigated by Pintner.[3] The ability to reproduce the meaning of what has been read is a further problem, one of the aspects of reading that is

[1] Hamilton, Francis, "The Perceptual Factors in Reading." "Archives of Psychology." Columbia Contributions to Philosophy and Psychology, 17, 1907.

[2] Huey, E. B., "The Psychology and Pedagogy of Reading ", 1908.

[3] Pintner, R., "Inner Speech during Silent Reading." Psychological Review, 1913.

measurable by tests. Of course, in order to reproduce what is read one must be able to grasp the thought conveyed by printed words, and this requires a background of experience whereby to interpret the ideas expressed. Inability to do this is quite a different matter from inability to master the mechanics of reading. For acquiring the latter, Meumann states that teaching should be adapted to the various types of children, among whom he includes those who, because of strongly fluctuating attention, have difficulty in eye fixation. Such children require formal practice to aid them in acquiring sharper visual impressions. Further differentiation of teaching method might be considered necessary for individuals who use different types of imagery — visual, auditory, and motor. However, since vision, audition, and motor processes are all involved in reading, Meumann believes that, practically, little heed need be given to imagery types.

The details of methods for teaching reading will not be entered into here; there has been much debate concerning the relative merits of the different procedures now in use. It should be recognized that discussion has been largely based on logical deductions and that little of either practice or theory in this field rests upon any scientific basis.

By way of summary, it may be said that analysis of the reading process shows that there are involved (a) perception of form and sound, and discrimination of forms and sounds; (b) association of sounds with visually perceived letters, of names with groups of symbols, and of meanings with groups of words; (c) memory, motor, visual, and auditory; and (d) the motor processes, as used in inner speech and in reading aloud. Reviewing the whole process, we see that in the actual performance of reading there must be finally some synthetic process uniting all the separate elements. This is a point that has been little emphasized by students of the psychology of reading, but its validity and importance seem clearly established through our analysis of cases of special difficulty in reading.[1]

Analysis of the mental processes involved in reading has never been applied to individual cases of inability to learn to read, so far as we know. The fact that some individuals have a pronounced disability in this field has been observed, it is true. It is exceedingly interesting to find that neurologists and even ophthalmologists have dealt with this question far more than have psychologists. It is the former who have reported and analyzed cases of so-called *congenital word-blindness* or *alexia*. Perhaps it would be best briefly to review the main contributions dealing with this subject.

Morgan[2] told in 1896 of a lad, fourteen years old, who, in spite of much instruction, could read only a few of the simplest words, could write almost nothing from dictation, and made mistakes even in writing his own name. He learned to read the letters of the alphabet only after long and painstaking instruction, but he had no difficulty in reading numerals. He solved simple problems in algebra and could multiply three-place digits. He came of an intelligent family, and except for his special disability was considered not inferior to others of his age. Morgan believed the inability to learn to read and to write from dictation was due to some congenital defect

---

[1] As early as 1896, Richard Baerwald in his book "Theorie der Begabung", discussing the psychology of reading, included the synthetic aspect. He calls synthesis in reading a mental function dealing with meanings of words and relationships of ideas whereby the content of a passage is grasped. He believes this synthetic process should be differentiated both from association and from apperception. However, we use synthesis to signify a process which binds together the separate elements in the mechanics of reading.

[2] Morgan, W. Pringle, "A Case of Congenital Word-Blindness.", *British Medical Journal*, November, 1896.

in the cortical center for visual memory of words and letters. Definite as his presentation of the case is in some aspects, there is no study of the various mental processes, not even of visual memory.

Following the publication of this article several English ophthalmologists became very much interested in the problem, and from that date up to the present time they have reported a number of cases brought to them for examination as possibly suffering from defective vision. Hinshelwood has offered a book on the subject [1] and several articles containing in all four case-studies: [2] (1) A boy of eleven could not read letters, words, or numerals, yet he remembered pictures, recognized them later, and had such good auditory memory that he learned his reading lessons verbatim. (2) A boy, ten years old, said to be bright and intelligent, could read numbers well, knew his letters, but could read only a very few words. (3) A girl of ten after four years in school could read the book of Standard I only with difficulty. It had required nine months' teaching before she could recognize the letters of the alphabet. She, too, had good auditory memory, could spell and write correctly even from dictation, and could add, subtract, and multiply. (4) A boy of seven attended school three years without having gained power to read. He could repeat the alphabet orally, but had trouble in recognizing the letters. Oral spelling was quite satisfactory, and he could read figures up to twenty. He was considered by his mother to be a bright boy. Three months after he was first seen he was reported to have made excellent progress; at that time he could read letters, the whole of the primer, and figures up to one

---

[1] Hinshelwood, James, "Letter-, Word-, and Mind-Blindness", 1902.
[2] Hinshelwood, James, "Congenital Word-Blindness", Lancet, May, 1900; "Congenital Word-Blindness", Ophthalmic Review, 1902.

hundred. This progress was attributed to training given him individually for several short periods a day. Hinshelwood states that where there is no ocular defect and no lack of general intelligence, the diagnosis in such cases must be that of congenital word-blindness. He concludes, on the basis of the above cases, that "visual memories of words, letters, and figures are deposited in different areas of the cerebral cortex." He advocates the use of blocks for training, developing thereby "muscle memories" to take the place of "visual memories."

Nettleship[1] reports a case of a boy of eleven who easily acquires information presented orally; he can pronounce words spelled to him and spells orally fairly well. He is fond of carpentry, plays games quite well, his vision is normal, yet he can read only a few words. Another boy, age not stated, reads music and draws well, but cannot read words. Details, even information concerning the educational opportunities, are not given. This author presents three other cases all similar to the above, one of which has been frequently cited because Nettleship reported that nine years after the first examination the patient had progressed to the point of reading fluently, and, indeed, had become a lawyer.

In 1904, Sidney Stephenson[2] described two cases: One, a boy of nine, was found to have good powers of observation and good visual memory; he could sketch the details of a machine or building. He reasoned well, but added to his great disability in spelling and reading was trouble with arithmetic. Six months later the boy's father stated that there had been improvement in both reading and arithmetic following individual instruction.

---

[1] Nettleship, E., "Cases of Congenital Word-Blindness or Inability to Learn to Read." *Ophthalmic Review*, 1901.
[2] Stephenson, Sidney, "Congenital Word-Blindness." *Lancet*, September, 1904,

Before further educational efforts could be made, the lad unfortunately died. The second case was that of a boy of ten who for five years had been the victim of extreme habit-spasm and likewise suffered from defective hearing and defective vision. Heredity was negative; mentally he was said to be "bright as a lark and sharp as a needle." He had good memory, learned easily, and retained well what he learned. His school grades in divinity, history, and geography were good. In arithmetic his work graded twenty per cent. He could not read either printed matter or handwriting; he could copy from the printed book, but writing from dictation was very poor.

Among later English writers may be mentioned C. J. Thomas.[1] This author apparently accepts as definitely localized, "Four special places in the cortex of the brain, which are known as speech-centers or word-centers. . . . These are the auditory speech-center, the visual speech-center, the motor speech-center, and the writing-center." In word-blindness it is the visual speech-center that is imperfect; "word memories cannot be made" and it is therefore difficult to learn to read, write, and spell. The cases discussed by Thomas indicate that he believes inability to write from dictation frequently involves defects in three of the speech-centers — auditory, visual, and writing. At other times the difficulty is due to imperfections or defect of "the associations between the visual speech-center and the writing-center." We do not know on what bases these conclusions rest.

In an earlier study [2] he cites seven cases all too briefly, without any record of tests, and exhibiting no new or uncommon features. But merely on the basis of ordinary

---

[1] Thomas, C. J., "The Aphasias of Childhood." *Public Health* (London), 1908.

[2] Thomas, C. J., "Congenital Word-Blindness and its Treatment", *Ophthalmoscope*, August, 1905.

observation, he makes the generalization that while visual memory for words may be very defective, visual memory for all else may be normal or even unusually good. He tells of a boy unable to read, who was nevertheless said to be a visualizer because his powers of observation and description were excellent. Another was said to have marvelous visual memory for objects.

In 1911, McCall[1] reported very briefly a case resembling those previously described by others, but designated by her an instance of congenital aphasia. More recently Whipham[2] gives in slightly more detail the case of an eight-year-old girl who cannot say the alphabet although she can write it perfectly on occasions. She cannot spell words of two syllables, cannot read even easy words, nor write from dictation. She can count to twenty and write numerals to twelve. She answers questions, obeys 'commands, has a good memory. She knows the days of the week, but not the months of the year. She has attended school for two years.

Besides the work of the English writers, some few other cases have appeared in various journals. Otto Wernicke[3] of Buenos Ayres tells of a girl of nineteen who seemed of normal intelligence; she spoke two languages, could read numbers correctly, but she could read printed matter only slowly and after spelling the words first. A boy of ten, whose father was alcoholic and whose older brother was feeble-minded, seemed lively and intelligent. He could read six-place numerals readily and could recognize geometrical figures. Letters were identified

[1] McCall, Eva, "Two Cases of Congenital Aphasia in Children." *British Medical Journal*, May, 1911.
[2] Whipham, T. R., "Congenital Word and Letter Blindness." *British Journal Children's Diseases*, Vol. 13, 1916.
[3] Wernicke, Otto, "Congenital Word-Blindness." *Centralblatt für Praktische Augenheilkunde*, September, 1903.

with difficulty and syllables or words not at all. Foerster [1] tells of a man twenty-seven years old, who could copy a text, but could not read or understand what he had written; he recognized the letters separately and even single syllables, but no words. He could write three numerals from dictation and could read numbers of four digits. However, it should be added that this subject was feeble-minded.

This case was discussed by Madame Dejerine, who believes the term word-blindness should be confined to the sense in which it is used by neurologists, namely, loss of ability to read and write due to cerebral lesion on the part of one who had previously been able to do so. She felt it unwise to confuse a *loss* of function with the *absence* of a function. Brissaud [2] and other French authorities concur in this view.

Indeed, this is the standpoint of practically all neurologists; they discuss the results that follow definitely localized cortical lesions. It is noteworthy that even C. Wernicke [3] in his classic article on disturbances of written language, makes no mention of congenital word-blindness. Ladd and Woodworth [4] define word-blindness or alexia as "inability to read, occurring, of course, in a person who previously could read and who has not become blind." The writing center, definitely localized by some and believed to be defective when there is difficulty in spelling and writing from dictation, they state has merely been

[1] Foerster, M. R., "A propos de la Pathologie de la Lecture et de L'Ecriture (Cécité Verbale Congénitale chez un debile). *Revue Neurologique*, 1904, p. 200.

[2] Brissaud, M., "Cécité Verbale Congénitale." *Revue Neurologique*, 1904, p. 101.

[3] Wernicke, C., "The Symptom-Complex of Aphasia: II. Disturbances of Written Language." Translated from "Die Deutsche Klinik" in "Diseases of the Nervous System", edited by Archibald Church, 1908.

[4] Ladd and Woodworth, "Elements of Physiological Psychology", 1911.

asserted, but "negative and mixed cases have sufficient weight to prevent a general acceptance of this localization."

A number of writers have discussed the etiology of this defect, some endeavoring to prove the thesis that heredity is a cause. Thomas [1] tells of a child whose mother said that she and five other children all were unable to learn to read. Stephenson [2] has reported a case where three generations were affected, the maternal grandmother, four of the mother's siblings, and the patient, a girl of fourteen. All the data were general reports, no one but the patient having personally been seen. Plate [3] writes even more unsatisfactorily of four cases in one family; the only peculiarity in these instances consists apparently in inability to spell correctly. Several other similar types of cases are reported. In general the facts of heredity in all the published studies are extremely inadequately known.

One of the best articles from the standpoint of review and discussion of the literature is presented by McCready.[4] He attempts to strengthen his thesis — "that there is distinct hereditary influence there can be little doubt" — by citing reported cases where the patient came of a neuropathic family. But without reconciliation to this view, he further adds as causes, defective intra-uterine development, injuries at birth, acute infectious diseases in infancy, and defective post-natal development. He gives a case which he calls congenital word-blindness, that was

[1] Thomas, C. J., "Congenital Word-Blindness and its Treatment." *Ophthalmoscope*, August, 1905.

[2] Stephenson, Sidney, "Six Cases of Congenital Word-Blindness Affecting Three Generations of one Family." *Ophthalmoscope*, August, 1907.

[3] Plate, Erich, "Vier Fälle von Kongenitaler Wortblindheit in einer Familie." *Muenchener Medizinische Wochenschrift*, August, 1909.

[4] McCready, E. B., "Congenital Word-Blindness as a Cause of Backwardness in School Children." *Pennsylvania Medical Journal*, January, 1910.

associated with stuttering. This is reported with only a meager psychological analysis and no record of tests.

Witmer,[1] using the term, *amnesia visualis verbalis*, reports the case of a boy, fourteen years old, whose abilities and disabilities were as follows: (1) general intelligence equal to or above the average; (2) ability to express thoughts in spoken language. normal; (3) memory for sounds good; (4) visual memory for color, simple geometrical forms, and separate letters good; (5) visual memory for words defective; he cannot read; (6) spells correctly only such words as can be spelled from component sounds. This boy was found to be suffering from severe diplopia, which Witmer believed had prevented the storing up of normal visual images. To this was due the inability to read and spell, rather than to congenital word-blindness.

The discussion to which this case led illustrates the need for differential psychological as well as physiological diagnosis. McCready thought Witmer's explanation insufficient; if the boy could draw well and possibly could recognize numerals (this latter point not having been specifically negated by Witmer), it would seem there was no general visual defect. In the analysis of the case, these specific facts are not covered nor are the tests given; one is therefore left in final doubt regarding the problem.

We have seen several instances where word images had not been accumulated, due to vision so defective as to preclude the possibility of acquiring clear visual pictures. We have not thought of interpreting such cases as due to an inherent disability for reading; the trouble is functional as far as the central nervous system is concerned, normal imagery having no chance for development.

Reviewing the work thus far done, it may be said that the English school first used the term congenital word-

[1] Witmer, Lightner, "A Case of Chronic Bad Spelling, *Amnesia Visualis Verbalis*." *Psychological Clinic*, August, 1907.

blindness and has offered most of the published cases. On the whole, from a psychological standpoint, these cases have been very inadequately studied and poorly analyzed; no psychological tests have been used, and no standard for gauging general intelligence has been employed. Tasks placed in the Binet scale at the four-year level of intelligence are cited as evidence of good mentality in the case of an eleven-year-old boy. Even visual memory has not often been tested. All together, the material is most unsatisfactory. Congenital defect of a visual word-center has not been proved or even recognized by neurologists. Indeed, the evidence in favor of a congenital defect localized in a definite visual center for words rests solely on the inability to read, an interpretation based on a supposed analogy to disabilities due to known cerebral lesions.

When we consider the complexity of the reading process and the various phases of mental life that are involved therein, we are led to wonder whether the phrase "congenital word-blindness" is anything more than a blanket term, easy to apply, but of little value either for understanding the problem or for offering help in regard to training. If inability to read can be due to inadequate functioning of other mental processes, such as the synthesizing faculty we have already dwelt on, there is left no support for the alleged fact of narrowly localized cerebral insufficiency, though this does not mean that some central defect does not exist. The definite criteria formulated for diagnosis, particularly by McCready, cannot be regarded as scientifically established. He states: "Given a child of school age, intelligent in other respects, not backward in other studies, who has difficulty in learning to read and who constantly makes mistakes, who has normal vision or refraction corrected by glasses, there should be no hesitancy in attributing the trouble to congenital word-blindness." At the present stage of our knowledge there is no establishing by symptoms the fact of congenital localized neural lesions or defects analogous to acquired lesions, and our case-histories show that inability to learn to read may rest upon a basis of various defective powers.

Though we agree with various authors in the fact itself, namely, that there sometimes does exist a special defect or disability in reading, yet in our own discussions, we have avoided the use of the term word-blindness. At the present time its use is questionable and much more experimentation is necessary in this field before other defects can be ruled out as possible explanations of disability for reading, alexia. In any case, there is no particular value in the term congenital word-blindness. What is needed in every case is study of all mental processes, careful, thorough, and of as wide a range as possible, with thoughtful analysis of the results — analysis which shall reveal not only the defective processes, but also the capacities that may be used as compensatory in training.

SPELLING

The problems of spelling will be only briefly discussed, for it is quite generally recognized that individuals differ widely in their ability to master this subject. All writers on the question have agreed that many persons well educated are unable to spell correctly. The studies of Rice [1] lead to the conclusion that the amount of time devoted to the teaching of spelling and the methods used have little correlation with the results achieved. He found that in various school systems the periods given for teaching spelling vary greatly, but that the results bear no relationship to this factor of time and drill. Methods of teaching used in this field are as yet little deter-

[1] Rice, J. M., "The Futility of the Spelling Grind." *The Forum*, Vol. 23, 1897.

mined by any psychological laws.   Lay [1] and Abbott and Kuhlmann [2] have studied experimentally the psychological elements involved in spelling, in an effort to find the success that follows auditory presentation of words as compared with visual, and to discover the differences when these processes are accompanied by soft and loud speaking and other motor reactions, such as the movement of the hand in writing the word.   Upon the whole, all studies emphasize the fact that discrimination of sound and association of visual form with the sound of the word are main elements in spelling.

In our own work we have never concerned ourselves much with any defect for spelling as such, that is, where no other difficulties in learning were found.   This attitude has been adopted because of the fact before stated, namely, that many intelligent and well-educated people remain all their lives poor spellers.   However, we have noted that poor spelling is often correlated with poor reading ability and at times with other disabilities in language.

SPOKEN LANGUAGE

The development of ability to use language as a medium of expression has been discussed by numerous writers. Kirkpatrick [3] believes that speech is an expressive instinct which owes its origin to other instincts.   The desire to express, to make wants known, begins with gesture and various cries; the latter, really vocal manipulations, develop into words through imitation coupled with the play instinct and encouraged by approval.   First mere sounds are made, then follows the period of "word-

[1] Lay, "Studien und Versuche über die Erlernung der Orthographie", 1908.
[2] Abbott and Kuhlmann, "On the Analysis of the Memory Consciousness." *Psychological Review*, Monograph Supplement XI, 1909.
[3] Kirkpatrick, E. A., "Fundamentals of Child Study", 1911.

learning" and later the sentence-making stage. Pronunciation is a matter of auditory perception coupled with memory and requiring control of voluntary musculature.[1]

Defect in ability to use language for purposes of self-expression is evidenced by poor vocabulary, wrong use of words, and incoherent statements as well as by special tests. The old notion that if one understood a fact or had an idea he could readily express it, is not altogether true. Sometimes one feels certain that there is an understanding, a comprehension, a thought, but that the expression of it is totally inadequate.

The term *congenital word-deafness*, referring to inability to understand and use spoken language, is frequently used, but few cases can be found in the literature. The condition is not often met and we have never studied a case in our own clinic.

Town [2] presents the only thoroughly studied case we find; that of a boy eight years old whose condition, however, was probably not congenital, but dated as early in life as the first week, when he had a serious illness accompanied by spasms which left him partially paralyzed on the left side. The paralysis disappeared during infancy. At sixteen months he contracted measles, which was followed by chorea, and at three years an attack of

---

[1] It is obvious that there may be extreme disabilities for language dependent upon brain lesions or brain defects, just as there may be cerebral motor paralyses. Cases of the type which Broadbent ("Cerebral Mechanism of Speech and Thought", *Medico Chirurgical Transactions*, Volume 55, February, 1872) first reported, where there was word-blindness with motor aphasia, have not been dealt with in this book. In our clinic we have seen a number of instances where it was plain that language disability was altogether disproportionate to the general intelligence; for instance, a young boy totally unable to speak very evidently understood directions given through signs. Although these are educational problems to some extent, they are so primarily neurological that they seem not in place in this volume.

[2] Town, Clara Harrison, "Congenital Aphasia." *The Psychological Clinic*, November, 1911.

scarlet fever left an otitis media. At the time of the examination he was well nourished and showed no lack of coördination in either eye or hand movements. He could not understand or use language normally, nevertheless he gave no evidence of general mental defect. He made his wants known by means of gestures and comprehended directions given him by signs. He understood the uses of objects, gave evidence of retentive memory, was interested in finding the causes of events, and quick to perceive visual stimuli of all kinds. Nor was he deaf to noises. He could repeat words uttered in an ordinary tone, not correctly, but in a way that approximated the original. He could name about thirty-six objects or their pictures and used voluntarily about twenty-four words, having in all a vocabulary of at least sixty words. On the other hand, he apparently understood only about twelve very simple words when spoken. He heard other words, as was proven by the fact that he would repeat them, but he did not understand them, as was shown by his failure to comply with requests or point out objects. On the Binet tests which were given him, he passed all the tests up to and including those for children of six years which did not require the understanding of language, failing in all those whose meaning could not be conveyed by gestures. Good visual perception of form was shown in his handling of the form-board test, which was done accurately and without hesitation. Color discrimination was good, and he showed some initiative in cutting from paper simple figures without aid or suggestion. The special diagnosis reached was that the boy was suffering from mental defect limited to the language field and independent of any other mental deficiency. The second case reported by Doctor Town is less thoroughly studied and is less convincing. In this instance, also, the child had suffered from otitis media.

In cases of this type every effort in determining etiology should be made to rule out abnormal conditions of the auditory apparatus as possible cause of ordinary auditory images not being stored. (This would make a situation similar to non-acquirement of normal visual impressions on account of defective eyesight.) An essential peculiarity in regard to this problem is that tests proving hearing normal at the time of examination by no means show that in the past there was no auditory defect, such as would be caused by an inflammatory process, notably otitis media. Lack of consideration of this important point reduces the value of the cases of "word-deafness" reported by Thomas [1] and McCall,[2] neither of whom gives developmental history to rule out any prior difficulty with the auditory apparatus. Also, curiously enough, both of these instances are given without any detailed study of the facts of general intelligence.

CASE STUDIES OF DEFECT IN LANGUAGE ABILITY

The examples given cover disability in learning to read and in use of language, incidentally including difficulties with spelling as they are correlated with other language defects.

Case 14. This case is presented as illustrating defect in special mental processes leading to disability for reading. Here we find a marked deficiency in auditory powers, shown by poor auditory memory and defective discrimination of sound. In marked contradistinction, other mental traits are normal or above normal.

Adolph J., 15½ years old, was sent to us as a behavior case, but proved to be much more an educational problem.

---

[1] Thomas, C. J., "Congenital Word-Blindness and Its Treatment." *Ophthalmoscope*, August, 1905.

[2] McCall, Eva, "Two Cases of Congenital Aphasia in Children." *British Medical Journal*, May, 1911.

We found him a most interesting study. In many ways the boy was exceedingly capable. He was American born and he had never been truant, yet after attending schools, both public and private, from his sixth year to his fifteenth, he was only in fifth grade. Still, as seen in the laboratory, he showed a splendid attitude toward mental tasks; he was greatly interested in all the tests and made an effort to do well. On the whole, he showed very good powers of attention and worked persistently with no evidence of fatigue. His emotions seemed altogether normal, both as seen in his reactions during the test work and as evidenced by his own and his mother's story.

Reading, no matter how simple the passage, occasioned him much difficulty. He made errors in the reading of very simple words, for example he called "often" "after", "about" was pronounced as "along." He failed absolutely on such words as "autumn", "winds", "frightened." Indeed, he never seemed certain of any words except the simplest, such as "the", "and", and other common monosyllables. Speaking of his reading, he said, "The kids at school would always laugh at me. I got so I wouldn't read at all. Sure, my teachers tried to help me, but it seemed like I couldn't pick it up." He had never read a book, could not read the newspapers, and, in consequence, was very poorly informed in spite of his good ability in many directions.

Turning to other school work, we found that the boy had no difficulty with arithmetic. He had had little opportunity of learning upper grade work, but was familiar with the fundamental processes and did quite well all tests involving money and its use, and also problems in arithmetic. On the other hand, spelling was exceedingly poor; we found that the boy could not depend upon the sound of words at all; these very evidently meant nothing to him. He himself said he had to learn his spelling entirely by "the looks of words." He eyed quite critically the word "gril" intended for "girl", and he finally decided that it looked all right. After writing the word "print" for "printer", he wanted to know if that really was "printer" or "painter", he thought he might have confused the two; he had no sense of the phonetic values.

Other test results brought out some very interesting features. All construction tests were done well, showing very good perception of form and form relationships. The method employed was planful and showed the boy to be rather deliberate and thoughtful in the solving of problems of this kind. As evidenced by several other tests, designed for the purpose, we found his perception of form and the discrimination of one form from another to be quite normal. Visual perceptions were accurate and rapid. Allowed to look at a picture for ten seconds, the boy gave details accurately, having noticed many of the minor points. Powers of analysis and mental representation were found to be distinctly good, tests in these fields being done very rapidly and with ease. General powers of apperception were extremely good. This was shown both on special tests for apperception and by his courtesy and other good general social behavior. The boy was exceedingly keen and quick in grasping the gist of a situation, in making inferences, and in the understanding of his own peculiar handicaps. Indeed, this characteristic and his good reasoning ability were very striking.

He demonstrated ability to analyze and reason, not only with concrete problems presented him, but in other fields. His quickness in replying to the common-sense tests of the Binet series, his keen sense of humor in the incongruities test, his good ability in arithmetic problems, all corroborated this. He was critical of his own performances, noting for himself any errors which he made and correcting them. Thus, after completing the continuous subtraction test, he said, "I made a mistake in that", and proceeded to correct his errors. In the description of pictures his excellent interpretations indicated splendid powers of imagination. His association processes were well controlled; verbal associations were extremely rapid. He showed normal learning ability in the forming of associations between arbitrary symbols. Psychomotor control was not particularly good, the boy being quite accurate, but slow in tests for this.

The study of the memory processes presented several points of great interest. Visual memory was at least normal both for rote and for logical material, but in the auditory field there were striking defects. In spite of his exceedingly good powers in other ways, this boy found the greatest difficulty in reproducing five numerals given him auditorily. He succeeded only once in twelve trials. This is a record much below the normal for his age; a five-place number should be readily reproduced by an eight-year-old child. In the passage for logical memory, presented to him auditorily, he did very well, but here he was aided by the ideas which he reproduced, as well as by the ability to transpose the auditory passage into visual terms. There were numerous verbal inaccuracies, and the English employed was exceedingly poor. Memory for syllables, given auditorily, likewise was much below normal; indeed, there were many evidences that this boy had a distinct defect in the auditory field. His enunciation was extremely faulty, though his vocabulary showed a fairly wide range. He was unable to reproduce catch sentences given him, such as "Thomas Theophilus Thinkum Thunkum", or "Round the rough and rugged rock the ragged rascal ran", even though these were repeated to him three times or more. He never succeeded in saying the word "Constantinople." It was evident that he did not hear all the sounds, for certain syllables were slurred over in every trial. In reciting a verse of "America", he enunciated many words poorly and used some incorrectly, for example, "Of Thee I See." He repeated this when the verse was said for him with the words very clearly enunciated. (It should be added here that physical examination showed no defect in hearing.)

In the light of the results on these tests, it is not so difficult to understand why this boy has been unable to learn to read. No doubt the clue is to be found in his defective auditory powers. His auditory perceptions are exceedingly faulty, and his auditory memory is very poor. Much of the help which comes consciously and unconsciously from the auditory field was lost to this boy. Remembering that both association of sounds with visual stimuli and auditory memory are elements in the reading process, there is no reason to doubt that defects in these functions may cause inability to learn to read.

Nothing had ever been done to help this boy overcome his handicap by adapting methods to his needs. Surely, since he can get certain sounds correctly and can speak so that he can be understood, even though his enunciation is poor, his auditory powers could have been improved by training. This would seem a justifiable deduction, but it does not mean that this could be done without special effort. To have used more extensively his naturally good visual powers might also have been a vast help.

It is quite clear how much this boy's time had been misused in the school, for with his very good ability in so many directions he could have progressed much more rapidly. To have spent nine years in the first five grades and even then not have gained ability to read simple passages, has been a great wrong. His failure was not to be explained by any physical handicap; though small, he was in good physical condition, nor were facts of heredity and developmental and environmental history significant.

The educational failure, in this case, has distinct relationship to the boy's delinquencies. He was reported as earlier mischievous in school, and, because of annoying girls, was suspended. Later, when working, he engaged in petty stealing, and finally, after dissatisfaction with his work, ran away from home.

Case 15. In contrast to the preceding case is this example of inability to learn to read correlated with extreme defect in the visual field, the auditory powers being quite normal.

James M., fifteen years old, was brought us by his parents as an educational problem. They said that he had never learned anything in school, that his teachers had tried to help him, unsuccessfully, and the parents had reached the conclusion that "he is just good for nothing and won't ever do anything in school."

Examination for ability in the ordinary school subjects showed that the boy's retardation was due to his inability to read. Number work was well done for the fifth grade which he had reached, and geographical knowledge was quite accurate, but it was seen at once that reading was the stumbling block. The word "cylinder" was pronounced "candle", "crib" was read as "club", "tunnel" as "turn." These were typical errors made throughout a fairly simple passage. James told us that he could not master reading; that he had never read a book, although he had enjoyed stories read to him by his mother.

Mental tests proved this boy to be exceedingly capable in some directions. He did problems involving the use of concrete material in a thoroughly planful manner, solving them quite rapidly. He showed good psychomotor control. Tests requiring powers of mental representation and analysis were done readily. The memory tests for logical material were likewise done quite well, as far as general results went, but certain peculiarities were noted. In the test where a passage is presented by auditory means, that is, where it was read to him, he reproduced ten of the twelve ideas with fair verbal accuracy and almost in correct order. On the other hand, when he himself read a passage, he read it slowly and with much trouble, later reproducing eighteen of the twenty ideas, but with many changes in logical sequence. When the reproduction was completed, the boy himself said, "I know part of it was wrong, it didn't sound right," after which he explained the method he had used. He stated, "I read each line over and then said it to myself ", for, he explained, he was unable to learn anything which he did not first hear.

The striking defect in powers of visualizing was quite apparent in another test for visual memory. Shown the two geometrical Binet figures for ten seconds and then asked to draw what he had seen, the boy made errors in both. After a second exposure he reproduced the figures correctly. In explanation of this he very clearly stated that he had been unable to visualize the figures, but had described the forms to himself, as it were, and followed his own description. It was interesting to note that in the first reproduction, where errors were made, this was due to the faulty description to himself of what he had seen. Thus, he said to himself, "There are three squares connected together with the two outside ones turned opposite each other. The second time I said to myself, the middle square had one side out." In each instance the reproduction which he drew corresponded to his unspoken verbal description.

If we try to explain this boy's disability in reading, we should say, in the light of the results on tests, that it is due to poor visual powers. He himself recognized the fact that he had to learn most things through sound. He said, in regard to spelling, in which he was fairly accurate, "I can learn to spell words if some one spells them out to me or if I spell them out to myself. I have to hear the sound of the words." This corroborates, of course, what the boy previously said when reproducing the memory passage given him visually. Clearly, visual material which cannot be recast into auditory form, or summarized in terms of ideas, is hard for this boy to control. In reading, naturally, it would be most difficult to convert all the pictures of various words into other than visual terms, hence the boy's great failure in this whole field. It is very certain that this case could not be used as argument that trouble in learning to read even when caused by visual difficulties is due to a defect in the hypothetical visual word-center.

What might have been done for this lad had his trouble been understood years earlier than it was, is difficult to know now, but there is not the slightest doubt that without recognition of his defect in visual memory and powers of visualization, he could not be properly taught. On the other hand, with an effort made to develop powers of visualizing and to adapt methods to meet his particular difficulties, he might have made much greater headway. From the fact that he had learned to read shorter words, those more commonly met, it is evident that the visual powers, while doubtless much below normal, must exist to some extent, and individual training probably could have increased them enormously. By good phonetic drill, associating the sound of letters and groups of letters with the visual form, the number of words which would have to be remembered as visual wholes would have been gradually decreased, and a tool given whereby the boy might have helped himself to a considerable extent. His naturally good auditory powers had not been as greatly used in connection with reading as they might have been. It is evident that this boy had not been taught reading by the phonetic methods which at the present time are common. In any case, no doubt, he would have needed individual help in order to progress at a normal rate in reading.

No physical trouble which could be considered a factor was found; there were no sensory defects. The boy was in rather poor general condition. He had grown rapidly and was somewhat under weight for his height. There was complaint of sick headaches earlier, but not for about two years previous to our seeing him. The intelligent mother could give no facts concerning heredity or developmental history that were significant.

James' very good ability in many ways had not served to make his educational advance normal. He was at least five years retarded in school, for which he had acquired a dislike; he had been truant to a moderate extent, extremely disobedient at home, and had once run away, but returned the following day of his own accord. His retardation in school had led to friction between the boy and the parents, who, though they were most anxious to give him a good education, had shown themselves quite helpless in the matter of how this was to be done.

Case 16. The next problem presented is of great interest, because the inability to master reading is so clear and definite, though psychological tests reveal little in explanation. The various mental processes, each tested separately, seem quite normal. In the light of this fact we are led to wonder whether in reading there is not involved some subtle synthetic process, which, at the present time, we have no means of studying, but defects of which, nevertheless, are of extreme significance. This case is presented without any pretense of solving the problem definitely. It affords a striking commentary on the limitations of our present knowledge. This does not militate, however, against the validity of finding special defect, nor against appreciation of its practical importance.

Walter Z. is a boy whom we have seen on numerous occasions, and whom we have come to know quite well. When first brought to the laboratory he was just eleven years old, and during the five years that have since elapsed, we have followed his career with much interest. When we first knew Walter, we found that he was unable to read a single word of English. The parents were foreign born, though the boy was born in the United States. Walter attended a foreign speaking school before we knew him, but soon after this he was sent to the Parental School, to which truants are committed. There he was kept for nine months, and some special attention was given him. After this long period we found, on reëxamination, that he had learned absolutely nothing in reading. He told us, with very evident sincerity, how eager he was to learn to read. He was conscious of his disability in this direction and had a thorough appreciation of the handicap that it was. He expressed a great desire to attend public school in order that he might try to make some headway in reading. During a later period of a few weeks, when we had this boy under observation, an effort was made to teach him the reading of very simple words, but it proved a failure. We found that when the boy was taught to recognize one simple word, for example "not", he was able to identify this same word whenever it occurred on the page, but he never succeeded in remembering more than one or two words at a time, or in putting them together so that he could read a full sentence. The net result of his intensive training was the ability to recognize a few simple words.[1]   In testing his writing and spelling, we found that he was able to write very well from the standpoint of legibility and letter formation, but he never succeeded in mastering spelling.   At the age of fourteen he could not spell the word "one" or "school", and he had learned to write his own name only with the greatest difficulty.

Because of his inability to profit by all the effort that both he and his teachers made, we studied this boy's mental processes with much care.   He did many things exceedingly well, among them tasks involving functions which one would believe very vital in the reading process itself.   He has very good visual powers; not only is his visual memory quite normal, but he has a distinct gift for drawing, a talent which he showed early.   Although he has never had any special instruction, he has always shown great love for this form of art and produces drawings which are remarkable for an untrained boy.   His hand-work — basketry and woodwork — is likewise very well done.

His memory powers for logical material, presented in either auditory or visual form, were normal too, and auditory rote memory tests conformed to norms for his age. Simple performances involving analysis and mental representation were correctly solved, but when these same processes were required in complex situations, the boy did poorly.   Although he remembered readily and recombined nine arbitrary symbols, each representing a letter, he was unable to perform a code test where exactly the same power is required, except that there are twenty-six symbols to recombine.

Walter made a very good record on all construction

[1] Though at the time we were studying this case the point did not occur to us, we have since wondered what part recognition memory plays in learning to read.   An experimental investigation of this problem might be well worth while.

tests; he was able to follow directions very well, remembering the various steps in a fairly long process. When last studied, we found the boy still graded normal by Binet tests, where he failed only in giving definitions of abstract terms. He showed normal control of verbal associations and no difficulty either in comprehension or use of language. We found that he perceived and discriminated form readily and that he could learn rapidly to associate one arbitrary symbol with another.

Physically, although poorly developed for his age, Walter was quite well nourished and had no sensory defects of any kind. Heredity, so far as we were able to learn, was negative. Nor was there anything of significance in the developmental history. Environmental conditions were unsatisfactory, inasmuch as the father was alcoholic, and the family poor; the home offered little in the way of mental satisfactions.

It does not require much imagination to realize the relationship between this boy's disabilities and his school and later career. At twelve years of age he was still in the first grade. At fourteen years he had been advanced to the second grade in an effort to encourage him, and a kind teacher who was interested in the boy was making an effort to aid him by special instruction, but by the ordinary school methods. His naturally good ability in other directions was being called into play very little, nor was he receiving any instruction along those lines wherein he might have profited greatly. From both points of view he was severely handicapped. No means were being found to help him at the point of his weakness, nor was he being given opportunities to develop his special talents. He was not even being taught a trade. He was merely plodding along in the ordinary schoolroom with well-intentioned teachers who were devoting special time to him, but in ways which offered little chance of success.

No doubt it would require much ingenuity to devise special methods for training this lad in reading and spelling, but from such an effort more knowledge of experimental pedagogy might be acquired, it would seem, than can be gained from many courses offered in universities. To allow the boy to progress as rapidly as he might in other subjects would necessitate a more flexible school system than we now have, but no case could present a clearer illustration of the need for just this kind of flexibility.

The dire social effects of an irrational and clumsy school system could hardly be found more clearly illustrated than in this case. Walter was first brought into court for running away from home and for truancy. A short time later he was sent to the Parental School; after his release from there, the boy was further truant, and was brought into court when he was found begging on the streets. From the boy's own account, he was virtually driven to this because he could not earn a livelihood in any legitimate way. When a little over fourteen he left school, utterly unprepared to meet the world or to find his place in our economic system. He had no trade training. His talent for drawing had not been developed. He could perhaps have been an errand boy had his inability to read not practically precluded this. His family was poor, his father out of work, and the children hungry, and with a really fine spirit the boy turned to begging, as the only means of contributing to the family support that he could think of. When last we heard of him, he was earning a small amount by scrubbing floors and dusting in a factory where there was little likelihood of his advancing to any more lucrative form of employment. Walter has been a victim of his own innate defects, but also of society's methods of dealing with some of its hampered members.

Case 17. In order to emphasize the problem presented in the previous illustration, another instance is cited, very similar in general characteristics, but where the details vary somewhat. Here, again, a boy is hampered with special disability in reading most difficult to account for on the basis of such tests as seem to have a relationship to the factors in reading.

Harold N., eleven years old, we learned to know quite well through his having remained for a long period awaiting adjustment of difficult family conditions. We were asked to see this boy because he was found to be exceedingly retarded in school. He has been repeatedly studied at intervals during two years.

He is a big, strong, well nourished lad, very pleasant, responsive, and eager to coöperate. He has never been a delinquent and now presents only, as far as we are concerned, an exceedingly interesting educational problem. Later the vocational aspects of his case will have to be considered. He makes a very favorable impression upon one; he talks well; is fairly well informed, considering his age and advantages; evidently remembers what he hears and sees; is anxious to acquire an education, and shows in general a very normal, boyish attitude toward the world.

In spite of this, Harold has been an out-and-out school failure. When originally seen he could not read a first-grade passage. He recognized only a few very simple words, such as "am" and "boy." As for writing words from dictation, we soon discovered the boy became greatly confused, though he made every effort to succeed. He volunteered to write "man", making it "nam", and the word "and", writing it "anj", but he wrote correctly the words "run" and "can." These four words composed his entire writing vocabulary, and these had been acquired, as he himself acknowledged, because his teacher had made him write them hundreds of times. A few days later the alphabet was written for him, and he was asked to write certain words that were spelled out to him, his task being to find the individual letters in the alphabet and to copy them. He wrote "l" for "t" and "j" for "y." (As will be seen later, this boy had no visual difficulties.) He read figures correctly.

Seen six months later, having attended school during the intervening period, he still was unable to read a first-grade passage. He made such errors as the following: he called the word "in" "with"; confused the words "am" and "can." At that time he could not write any sentence, either from dictation or of his own invention. He could write just four words besides his name. A month later, during which time intensive individual help was given him, he did no better than before; indeed, he confused words which were being taught him with the few words that he had previously known. It should be added, however, that while given individual instruction by a very conscientious teacher, no specially adapted method was used. An effort was made to teach him by the usual means employed in teaching children who have no special disability.

For number work, we are not sure that there was any innate defect. Because of his having remained so long in the first grade he had had very little training in this direction, but concrete problems he did quite well; he added simple number combinations, added money correctly, solved very simple problems, such as, If nine apples are divided among three children, how many would each receive? But he could not tell abstractly one third of nine. We judged, on the basis of our test work, that Harold could learn numbers fairly readily if he had the opportunity of doing so. It is clear that his number ability, at least, is very far ahead of his reading ability.

This boy did exceedingly well on tests for general intelligence, such as the Binet tests. Here he graded above his age. He did the Binet test for visual memory very well; very quickly detected the Binet language incongruities and gave shrewd and relevant answers in the Binet common-sense tests. We found normal powers of apperception, both through special testing and judging by his conversation. He also demonstrated normal control of verbal associations and also normal ability to form such new associations as are required in the arbitrary learning test.

Harold proved on construction tests to be a rather thoughtful, deliberate boy, solving problems of this sort in a logical manner, with some trial and error, and profiting very quickly by his own experience. He did not repeat his errors and having once reached a solution, he remembered it and was able to solve the same problem on second trial with a very great gain in speed and accuracy. His powers of analysis and mental representation, as judged by our usual tests, were quite good. As for memory tests, we found immediate memory to be very good; memory span for rote material was just about what is expected at his age, neither better nor worse; memory for logical material read to him was not particularly good — he gave seven items out of a possible twelve; remote memory for this type of material was almost as good as immediate, for after forty-eight hours he reproduced six of the twelve items. It should be added that these represented the main ideas of the passage. On the Aussage, or testimony test, he gave a full coherent account, showing good and rapid perceptions, good powers of interpretation, and good memory. This last was further shown when, one year later, without having seen the picture again, he gave a detailed, accurate description.

He had great skill in handwork, showing more than average ability in this direction; his eye for line and measurement was accurate, and he evidenced quite a little artistic feeling for form. His manual training teacher considered him exceedingly capable in this work, saying the boy showed initiative and ability to plan. His success in this work and on tests indicated that powers of perception were in these fields unusually good.

What can we find peculiar in the mental processes to account for the boy's inability to learn to spell and to read? Studied separately, there is no difficulty or peculiarity or lack of functioning of any of the mental processes tested. Visual and auditory powers seem normal; in memory tests he reaches the norm for his age; association tests give no evidence of irregularity; there is no defect for language. Here again, as in the preceding case, one would like to know more about the general facts of recognition memory as involved in the reading process.

Nor was there any other explanation found. The boy has always been strong. He has been examined by various specialists, and the physical conditions can be ruled out' as being negative. We know the heredity and family history quite well in this case, and though there is much of interest, there is nothing that is directly significant in relation to the boy's disability. In spite of poor home conditions, Harold has attended school regularly and has had the same educational advantages that fall to the lot of most city boys.

Harold is still too young for us to appreciate all the social consequences that may arise as a result of his disabilities. He has as yet shown no delinquent tendencies, and placed on a farm where his defects are not strikingly apparent, he has been happy and has gotten along very well. His particular handicaps should be remembered, however, in all future efforts in his behalf.

Case 18. To show how impossible it is to analyze and explain reading defect if insufficient study is given, we cite the following instance in which the problem as presented to us was merely to determine whether the individual was normal mentally or feeble-minded. Unlike the previous illustrations, we have here insufficient data for ruling out the several possible explanatory factors.

Richard T., 16½ years old, had only reached the fourth grade of the public school when he left at fourteen years. He was considered a school failure, and because of this a number of people regarded him as being subnormal.

When he was tested for mentality, we wondered why he should be accounted so dull, for he did many things very well. We soon saw that the boy had a special disability for reading. He did performance tests normally, made a good record on tests for mental representation and analysis, had a normal record on tests for apperception, and while he had not had training in arithmetic above the fourth grade, he could add, subtract, and multiply. He had no difficulty in handling money or in solving simple problems involving money. On the other hand, his reading was exceedingly poor. He failed on all but the simplest words, and even these were read in a very hesitating manner, with much uncertainty. He himself told us that he had always had a great deal of trouble in school on account of his reading. From the results on tests given him, we were sure that the boy could not be regarded as anything other than normal in general ability, but we were unable to study his mental processes in sufficient detail to find out the explanation of his disability, though the fact that it existed was quite clear.

He was an extreme delinquent, having been in court numerous times for truancy, for stealing, and for not working. He was American born, but of foreign parentage. The family was poor; he was the only one of six children who had caused any trouble; all of the others had good school records; a sister of twelve was in the seventh grade. The father was said to have had fair intelligence and some education. The mother seemed on the whole quite dull, but she had had very poor educational opportunities.

How large a factor his special defect was in his delinquency we cannot say with surety, but, beyond doubt, it played quite a part; indeed, we are inclined to believe that it was a matter of very great consequence, since he early became a truant. School offered him no satisfactions, and when he left, at fourteen, he had little preparation for any particular vocation. We know that he had positions requiring practically no skill; for a time he worked with a peddler. The father had died when the boy was about fourteen, and there was poverty and poor parental control, and very little in the way of home interests. Had the boy been trained for some vocation which interested him it is quite conceivable that his whole career might have been very different.

Case 19. The following case illustrates defects in *general language ability* and the serious consequences that arise therefrom.

Thomas S., 15 years old, was in a room for subnormal children when we first knew him and had been held there for the past several years. He was tested on two different occasions, because when first seen he was apprehensive, ill at ease, and hence unable to do his best. Taking into consideration the boy's attitude and judging him by his best efforts, we found he did fairly well on tests for general ability. He himself told us, and testing corroborated it, that he was held in the subnormal room because of his inability to progress in reading. He could read only the most familiar monosyllables, he failed on all longer words and even on short ones when they were in the least unfamiliar. Nor was his achievement in writing much better. He wrote legibly, but could spell only very few words. He could add, subtract, and multiply, not a poor record considering that his opportunities for acquiring knowledge in arithmetic had been extremely limited.

On performance tests the boy did very well. All construction tests were solved correctly; good powers of motor control were shown; he succeeded where analysis and mental representation were demanded; he made a perfect record on the substitution learning test; and succeeded very well on tests for memory, so far as repetition of ideas was concerned. The notable feature here was the fact that although he could give a good reproduction of the thought of the passage read to him, yet his power of expressing the ideas was decidedly limited.

It was in the field of language that this boy's special disability lay. He could not express himself with force or accuracy; his choice of English was poor, even considering his home disadvantages. His parents were German, and their native language was spoken in the home. That the boy did not speak grammatically was perhaps not of any significance, but much more striking was it that he could not write, speak, or read German any better than English.

When the tests were analyzed, it was seen that this boy had normal powers of perception, both for form and relationships of form ; he reasoned quite well, at least in regard to situations presented concretely; apperceptions and memory were normal. On the other hand, the opposites test, which involves control of association of words, was performed very poorly and corroborated the findings in regard to other language factors. Thus, it can be seen that inability to learn to read was due, very likely, to a defect for language in general. No defect in visual or auditory fields was shown, nor in powers of forming new associations, that is, in actual learning capacity.

Physical factors could be ruled out, since examination showed the boy to be unusually strong for his age, with no sensory defects. Heredity and developmental conditions were likewise negative. Because of his one disability, regardless of what he could do in other tasks, the boy had been kept in the subnormal room. He himself said, "When I was in that room I could never get out and get pushed up. I know my numbers, and everything, excepting reading. Everything I did in woodwork was good, I made baskets and everything, but because I could not read I was kept down with the dippy ones." In spite of having been regarded by the school authorities as a mental defective, we could not so classify him in the light of results on tests, nor, indeed, according to his social reactions.

We note that when he left school shortly after our study of him, he was quite successful vocationally. Fortunately, his work was of such a character that his disability did not handicap him; he became a good wage earner, and so far as we know now, five years after our first knowledge of this boy, he has never again been delinquent in any way.

One interesting feature was found when the boy came to visit us, after having left school for several months. He had endeavored by himself to make some headway in reading and spelling, with greater success than had been accomplished in the school. It is true his achievement was very limited, he could not read all the words of a first-grade passage, but he said that by dint of much perseverance he had added some few words to his reading vocabulary. Certain it is that the school had been an utter failure in discovering the defect which was the basis of his lack of progress, and his own clumsy efforts were succeeding quite as well, if not better, than the methods used in school.

Case 20. Another example of general language disability is here presented.

Rupert N., sixteen years when first seen, was found at

once to be most peculiar. He was a great problem from the standpoint of conduct when we first became acquainted with him, and previously he had been an educational problem as well. Every one who came in contact with the boy felt him to be a peculiar, dull, loutish fellow. He made the most unfavorable impression, even in the court-room, because of his slouchiness and his confused and almost incoherent statements.

We soon found that very little reliance could be put upon any statements made by the boy himself. He was contradictory in what he said, and at all times seemed unable to give a clear and cogent story, even of his own actions. Both with us and at court his statements varied from day to day and from one hour to the next. He said that though he had gone to school for eight years, he did not learn much because his teachers were "no good", and only one of them ever taught him anything.

We have studied this boy over quite a long period of time in an effort to learn just what his native ability is. Mentally we have found him most peculiar, and after frequent examinations we have concluded that he is a border line type. He cannot be regarded simply as out-and-out feeble-minded, nor, on the other hand, can we regard him as altogether normal mentally. A number of things he does very well, but his disabilities are equally as apparent. His reactions, on the whole, are rather slow, except when working with concrete material.

In regard to his failures, the striking defect in several aspects of language ability was soon noted. We were impressed over and over again with the fact that words seemed to have no significance to this boy. He had the greatest trouble in expressing himself, nor could he control his verbal associations on tests requiring these. He made eight errors in giving the opposites to twenty simple words, a record that is extremely poor. Even when the correct reply was made, it required a very much longer time to think of the word than is normal. It was evidently language that had retarded this boy in school work, for his ability in arithmetic was far beyond that in spelling and reading. He knew all the fundamental processes, although he was not altogether accurate in the use of them, his mistakes being matters of carelessness. He was unable to write a simple sentence from dictation, and when he himself wished to write an account of his schooling, the result was ludicrous. Even very simple words were misspelled, as is shown in the following: "I neear wast ene plaes atsed in Chicago." (I never went any place outside of Chicago.)

On certain tests he did very much better, attaining records that were normal or very nearly so. Tests with concrete material he did very well, even those involving quite a little reasoning. His perception of relationships of form seemed quite normal; indeed, his records are rather above the average. Then, too, he seemed to have extremely good powers of visualizing; wherever this could be called into play, the test results were excellent. This was a notable factor which aided his performing correctly several of the more difficult tests. His results on tests for apperception, where these dealt with material presented in pictorial form, were normal; a result in contradiction to his social apperceptions, as shown by his conversation and behavior. Tests for mental control were not easy for him; he had much difficulty in keeping his mind on the task at hand, and his reactions here were very slow. As graded for intelligence by the Binet scale, he lacked one point of completing the twelve-year series. The interesting feature here was the fact that on first trial he failed on many of the tests which involved the use of language. He had much difficulty in incorporating words into a sentence or in rearranging words to form a sentence. In the latter task he never succeeded.

Analyzing the successes and failures, we find he had great difficulty in all work that deals with language; how much allowance should be made for this in evaluating the final score on the Binet scale is practically quite important if one uses this as the criterion for mental classification. Even more important, practically, is the influence of this special defect on school attainment, for no doubt without recognition of such a weakness, much school work is so poorly performed that the pupil becomes greatly retarded. More important still is the effect of such a handicap in vocational and social life. While certain occupations do not require the use of language, yet the inability to express oneself in regard to activities that deal with the most concrete material gives an impression of extreme stupidity and mental dullness. Perhaps, too, it impairs the ability of the individual himself to apperceive his relations to the world, if he is unable to express even to himself general principles. In the case of this boy there were, of course, other points to be considered before concluding that a special defect for language existed.

His parents were foreign born, and though a foreign language was spoken in the home at times, yet both the mother and father spoke English fairly well. The boy himself was born in this country and had always attended English-speaking schools. A brother, several years older, had progressed satisfactorily in school, entering the ministry later. From the parents' account of conditions, we found that heredity as well as the developmental history was negative. When Rupert was five years old he met with an accident in which his head was hurt, but he was not known to be badly injured and was not unconscious. No other point of significance was learned. The father, who seemed to be a thoroughly good, hard-working man, not well educated, but fairly intelligent, told us that this boy had always been a lazy fellow, never fond of school, and had had difficulty in learning, particularly reading.

Physical examination showed Rupert to be a large, strong lad, in very good general condition. Except for a rather dull expression, nothing of any significance was noted.

Some element of mental dullness was due, no doubt, to indulgence in masturbation, which the boy acknowledged, and this, of course, may have accounted for the slowness of mental reactions.

Naturally, at our institute, the question of a psychosis in this case has been considered over and over again. Dementia has been pretty surely ruled out because of the boy's good control of his mental processes in some respects at all times. Then he has shown definite improvement on several types of tests when reëxamined at a considerable interval. He did better on Binet tests, on continuous subtraction, and on the association test for opposites, where a better score was made for time and accuracy.

His delinquencies, which consisted of running away from home, long periods of idleness, during which he has loafed about and become involved in stealing and burglary, may be partly explained by his laziness due to bad sex habits, possibly by the influence of adolescence, and by bad companionship, the latter factor accentuated by the lad's social suggestibility. Aside from all these forces, however, the boy presents a problem difficult to adjust because of his peculiar mental make-up which cannot be altogether disregarded in any constructive efforts undertaken in his behalf. That he has special abilities in working with concrete material and in visual powers, that he has, likewise, quite a specialized disability, as shown in all tasks requiring the use of language, is of practical significance in determining his future, just as it has been an element in the causations that explain his past failures, educationally and vocationally. Since he has had the usual opportunities for acquiring an ordinary vocabulary and for using it, and yet has not succeeded in so doing, we are led to conclude that there is an innate defect of a highly specialized nature.

CHAPTER VII

Special Defects in Separate Mental Processes

Sometimes one finds in the course of a psychological examination certain defects of some one or more of the mental processes which, though having an important influence on achievement, are not correlated with learning the school subjects which have already been discussed. Their existence and relationship to the school and social career may be unsuspected because, unlike instances of reading or language defect, no incapacity for some one kind of learning is found. Rather, there may be some general disability in mental functioning which affects all work, making the individual unusual in his reactions. Such defects in mental processes are often the explanation of failures that seem inexplicable. Hence, it is of very great value to discover defects of this character and to determine their practical significance.

Following are presented some types of defective functioning of mental processes which, experience has shown, have important bearings.

DEFECTS OF MEMORY

Memory is a function that presents varied phases, all of which might be discussed, for defect may possibly be found in any one and not exist in others. The term memory is used in everyday speech with different meanings; and experimental psychology has investigated quite a number of problems dealing with this mental process. There are studies of recall and of recognition; of immediate and remote memory; of memory for different kinds of material, for sense perceptions, symbols, products of ideational processes, and for emotions. There are studies, too, of memory for logical and for rote material; for visual, auditory, or motor percepts.

The relationships of these aspects of memory to each other and applications to complex activities are not altogether known. It has already been stated in a previous chapter that experimentation directed towards determining the degree of correlation that exists between different phases of memory has led to the general conclusion that there is a positive relationship of quite high degree. But such studies deal with very highly specialized processes; for example, the correlation between memory for words and memory for numbers, or between memory after one minute and memory after one hour.

Very many practically important laws of memory have not yet been determined; those most firmly established concern themselves mainly with nonsense or other types of material quite unlike the activities of everyday life. To what extent these laws obtain in applied fields we do not know. In a common-sense way, we are aware, of course, that in practical affairs both immediate and remote memory are essential, that we need to remember what we see and what we hear, that to remember ideas is probably more useful, in general, than to have a good memory for rote material, but that a defect for the latter may be of great significance in some kinds of school work, as well as in certain occupations.

It is perhaps unnecessary to give illustrative cases of peculiarities or defects in all these aspects of memory; in preceding case-histories many of them have been mentioned, and further mention will be made in case-histories that follow. It has been shown that some individuals have defects for auditory presentations; others for visual. It is true that persons of good intelligence frequently are not hampered by a defect for one or more types of memory; indeed, they may even be unaware that it exists, for defect in one field often is compensated by substitution in another field. Little is known as yet of the relationship of some phases of memory to learning school subjects, and especially it might be of great interest and value to study the rôle of recognition memory in reading.

To illustrate how widely ability in memory may vary in one field, two cases are cited, one of great disability and one of unusual ability in auditory rote memory.

Case 21. Henry J., 16 years old, was seen after he had been in court on several occasions. The mental examination proved interesting because it showed that the boy was quite intelligent and in general capable, but had a very specialized defect. The striking feature of all the test work with this boy was the finding that he was far below normal for his age in the matter of rote memory. When a series of numerals was presented to him auditorily he could not remember more than four. A memory span for five numerals is expected of normal eight-year-old children, but this boy failed to reach this standard, though given numerous trials. His memory span for numerals presented visually was not much better. He succeeded here with five. Memory span for syllables was likewise poor; the best record he was able to make was repetition of fourteen syllables. On the other hand, where ideas were to be recalled, that is, where memory tests dealt with logical material, the results were good. A passage presented auditorily and containing twelve items was reproduced with the omission of only one, and with fair verbal accuracy. The result on a logical passage which he himself read was not so good; he gave fifteen out of twenty ideas, though it should be added that his version included the principal ideas.

In many ways he showed more ability than the average boy of his nationality and social status. He was foreign born, but had come to this country when a very small child. The native language was spoken in the home and likewise in the school which the boy had attended during the greater part of his school career. He spoke English well, showed very good apperceptions in regard to his own home situation and his relationship to it, and did a number of mental tests very well. In spite of what one often finds in such cases, namely too little familiarity with English to do well on Binet tests where language is so largely involved, Henry passed well all the tests for ten years and all for twelve years, except the definition of abstract terms. Construction tests were very well solved and so were those involving analysis and mental representation. Association processes dealing with words were normal. School work was done sufficiently well to feel that no especial peculiarity or difficulty in regard to this existed.

We find here, then, a boy who shows by his general reactions and the results on many tests that he is quite capable, but who, nevertheless, has an astonishingly grave defect in certain of the memory processes. That this had not interfered more with his progress in school and his acquisitions on the basis of general world experience, is possibly due to the type of the disability and possibly to compensation. Nevertheless, in certain practical ways it might interfere with his vocational pursuits. Thus, in an effort to show the practical significance of his defect, we asked the boy to find in the telephone directory two telephone numbers, representing the different departments in the same firm, or the business and residence telephone numbers of some individual, and then after giving him a fair amount of time in which to learn them he was asked to repeat them. Although he tried very hard in this, he never succeeded in any one of a number of trials. Such a difficulty as this would preclude the possibility of success in office work, or, indeed, for any occupation where rote memory had to be depended upon.

His delinquency, staying away from home, was largely accounted for by home conditions, which were so wretched as to offer little that would satisfy any normal boy. The father was a very abusive and ill-tempered man.

Physically Henry was quite poorly developed for his age. He was small and not well nourished, but he was a bright-eyed, healthy looking boy, nevertheless. There were no sensory defects, nor was any history of severe illness obtained.

Case 22. Let us now contrast with the above case that of Benjamin L., a young man of over 20. He had had unusually fine educational opportunities, both from the standpoint of schools he had attended and the environment in which he lived. His family were well educated and cultured people, and since this boy was very companionable with both parents, he had, of course, gained much from the home surroundings. In spite of the chance for good mental interests, he did not care for book learning and had no desire to attend college. After leaving school he had been placed in a bank where he had to work largely with numbers.

Mental examination showed that this young man had certain very distinct abilities, the most striking of which was memory for rote material. For auditory presentations his record was twelve numerals correct, and thirteen were repeated with the transposition of only one numeral.

This remarkable performance was consistently maintained on several trials. For syllables, — that is sentences, but where there was no logical connection, — the record was likewise extremely good, thirty-two syllables being repeated without any effort. Other points brought out by psychological study were the following: He proved to have very good mechanical ability, handling concrete material with splendid perceptions and much skill. Likewise he possessed excellent ability in the use of language. He talked very well, showed a good discrimination in the choice of words and had a distinct gift for clear and effective presentation of his ideas.

None of the qualities in which he really excelled was being used in his vocational pursuits, whereas he was occupied with just the things that had always interested him least. We merely mention this as evidence of the fact that even in intelligent families there is little realization of talent and of weakness in the placing of young people in occupations.

There was not the slightest evidence that the training received by this young man accounted in any way for his unusually good rote memory, nor in the preceding case had education bettered innately poor memory span.

Case 23. Exceedingly defective remote memory may be found in an individual whose immediate memory is normal. This fact is clearly shown in the analysis of the following case, which illustrates likewise the practical significance of such a defect.

Peter R., 11 years old when first seen by us, has been examined many times during the year which has intervened since the first study. He has been tested by three examiners and retested by two of them several times. The mental characteristics which have been noted in the laboratory are quite in accord with the observations of his teachers.

On psychological examination it is apparent at once that there is no difficulty with immediate memory; a large number of varied tests all offer proof of this fact. That immediate visual memory is not defective is shown by the excellent results on the Binet figures and by his recital on the Aussage test. In the latter, after seeing the picture for ten seconds, Peter enumerated as many objects and details as are given by the average person of his age, and on cross-examination we found that he could give correct replies concerning many other items. For auditory stimuli immediate memory was also normal. Tests here were quite in accord with norms for his age. He could repeat five numerals readily, and occasionally six; in memory for syllables he did rather better than the norm, while auditory memory for logical verbal material proved to be very good. He formed new associations such as are required in the arbitrary association test; remembered directions told him orally, and was able to carry in mind and later imitate a series of movements involving six steps (the Knox Cube test), after having been shown three times; he could even remember and control four numerals presented auditorily when he was required to retell them backwards.

On a number of tests requiring very little memory and meant to gauge specifically other mental processes, he did very well. The construction tests were performed normally; both cross line tests were correct on first trial; the pictorial completion test was done well, and control of verbal association as indicated by the opposites test presented no unusual features.

What has impressed every one is the fact that this boy cannot retain for any length of time what he is able to learn immediately and what has been presented to him with most patient and persistent efforts. When we first saw him we were told that both his mother and his school teachers considered him a very dull lad. It was quite true that he had gained very little from all his school experience; he could not read a simple first-grade passage, and he could write only his name and three or four other words; adding simple number combinations constituted his acquirements in arithmetic. His writing is poor, the letters often are not properly formed; he is not only left-handed, but writes in an awkward, overhand fashion.

Since our first examination we know that the boy has attended the public schools for some five or six months, and that later he has received intensive and individual help during a period of four months by a teacher who has been most zealous in her efforts to help the boy. In spite of this, we find that he has made absolutely no headway in any of the school branches. He cannot remember the phonetic values of the different letters, although he has received a great amount of drill in these. At the end of a day's lesson he knows them, but by the next day they are forgotten. In consequence, he has made no progress in either reading or spelling.

For days at a time he has been drilled in the process of subtraction, and although he understands it and immediately after being taught can solve problems without error, yet when the drill is stopped for two or three days, all that he has learned has been absolutely lost. He knows a few of the simpler combinations of the multiplication tables; the more difficult ones he cannot remember. After he has been told the date again and again, if a few days elapse before he is questioned, he will make the wildest guesses; thus, after having heard each morning for several weeks that the current month was September, when the drill was stopped for three days he said in reply to a question that it was February. After months of effort he is finally able to name the months of the year without error, but he cannot remember his birthday or learn to tell time, and he acquires almost no information about events of the day. We are told that several of his schoolmates have endeavored to teach him, and that his responses to questions after an interval of some days are so ludicrous and his information is so absurdly confused that they roar with laughter at his errors.

The defect found by the above tests is corroborated by other tests for remote memory. He is unable to remember the figures of the arbitrary association test which he has done three times previously. He cannot recall the passage used in the auditory verbal test for logical memory; he does not remember that this test was given him the year before, although at the time the immediate reproduction was excellent. He cannot recall a single one of any of the short incidents used in the absurdities tests. When asked to describe any of the tests given to him previously, he is unable to do so. Trying to recollect the Binet test for three words in a sentence, he gives one of the three words incorrectly, although he had done the test well less than a month earlier. Very curious was his attempt to draw a simple scheme of the arrangement of three large buildings at an institution where he spent ten happy days some two months before. It seemed incredible that the relationships of the buildings should not have been recollected; he pictured them absurdly misplaced. Questioned about evening entertainments which have been given once a week at the institution where he is living, he tells us vaguely about stereopticon pictures of snow mountains, but cannot tell what country they are in nor can he recollect certain pictures of London, seen on another occasion, except to say that they were pictures of buildings in some old country.

It should be stated that this boy is a very faithful and industrious worker. He has been making the most serious attempts to take advantage of the efforts that are being made in his behalf. He will invent problems and bring them to his teacher when his routine work is completed. In the manual training room, although he shows some little initiative and good imitative ability, directions have to be given him over and over again.

Binet tests offer little that is of any help in interpretation of such a case; they do not indicate the particular defect which is the most interesting feature of the boy's mentality. The first record graded him 9¾ years mentally. His last testing, over a year later, indicated very little advancement; he has now learned the months of the year and succeeds on one other test previously a failure. Naturally, remote memory is so important an aspect of mental life that great disability in it affects learning to such an extent that an individual with this defect must be considered educationally and socially a defective. In the case outlined above we have always felt the prognosis to be poor; the boy will continue to grade as a moron.

The contrast between remote and immediate memory powers in this case is strikingly shown in the graphic form which we sometimes use in evaluating test results and we therefore append it:

TESTS FOR REMOTE MEMORY

Below normal	*Normal or above*
Visual memory	
Logical verbal memory	
General information	
Number work; processes and combinations	

Learning — as of birthday, date,
  current month, months of
  year, etc.
Reading, either by word pictures or phonetic values
Telling time
Relating past events

TESTS FOR IMMEDIATE MEMORY

Visual — Binet and other
  geometrical figures
Syllables — 24 correct
Memory span — 5 numerals
  always; 6 numerals oc-
  casionally
4 digits backwards
8 memories (Terman test
  read to him)
Substitution test
Auditory — verbal memory
  test
Aussage picture test
Knox Cube test — imitating
  a series of movements
Learning — as of school subjects, birthday, date, etc.

DEFECTS OF INNER VISUAL FUNCTIONS

Analogous to auditory defect, illustrations of defect
in visual functions are presented. No doubt such disability may be more or less specialized, the significance
increasing with the extent and degree to which the defect
exists. Certain of the practical correlations of visual
defects have already been noted in the discussion of dis-

ability for reading; but they are by no means limited to this school subject. They influence a much wider range of activities.

This type of disability is properly placed after memory defect because in considering defects in the visual powers, memory plays so large a part.

Case 24. Harry R., 14 years and 9 months of age, had made much slower progress in school than any other member of his large family. The boy was said to study hard at home, where the father and an older sister helped him frequently with his lessons. He was in the sixth grade, but maintained his position there only with difficulty. Although his family regarded him as retarded in school work, they considered him normal in all other respects. He was so conscious of his disabilities that he had become sensitive to the extent of crying bitterly if scolded because of his poor record.

Psychological examination showed that this boy's abilities were quite uneven, and that he had a striking defect in visual powers. His perception of form evidently was not notably poor, but perception of relationships of form was exceedingly defective. He failed to solve the simpler construction test, ordinarily performed by normal eight-year-old children. His efforts on the more difficult one were purely random; many impossibilities were tried, and the final result was likewise a failure. Visual memory was equally as defective. The Binet test for memory of geometrical figures was reproduced so poorly that the forms were altogether unrecognizable. A figure even simpler than either of the Binet forms was not reproduced correctly. Indeed, the boy failed on three or four tests all designed for testing visual memory. Neither could he draw the simplest diagram of the façade of his own house; after representing it by an oblong, he could not place the doors and windows.

In an attempt to draw the floor plan of his home he became utterly confused; he could not indicate where the doorway was located, nor how the rooms were arranged.

It was evident on the cross-line tests that the boy could not represent to himself the figures and the various parts, although he could draw the figures and number them correctly; even with the model before him he could not identify the sections. Clearly, his powers of visual representation were very defective. Associations between numbers and symbols as required in the substitution test were very slowly formed, the boy making on the whole a very poor record here. We noted on the apperception test that while he readily grasped the meaning of the situations depicted, he was slow in finding the pieces which he wished to insert. Indeed, wherever visual powers were concerned, the boy was slow and frequently unsuccessful.

In marked contrast to his poor visual powers, we found unusually prompt reactions to auditory stimuli. Memory span for numerals presented auditorily was beyond the norm for his age; he was able to reproduce eight digits with ease. Incidentally, we were interested in the fact that he repeated the numbers in phonographic fashion quite without effort. Memory for logical material where the passage was read to him proved to be very good, ten out of twelve items being given and these including the main ideas. Here the verbal accuracy was distinctly good. He did not do quite as well in the memory passage which he himself read; twelve of twenty items were reproduced in correct sequence, but we noted by the movements of his lips that the boy was saying to himself the words as he read them. Nor did there seem to be any difficulty in control of verbal associations; in the opposites test there were no errors or failures. Very good auditory discrimination was shown in repeating difficult sentences and phrases. Enunciation was good, and even catch phrases were repeated correctly. He sang "America" accurately.

General intelligence, as gauged by the Binet tests, was not defective; he graded through twelve years. He failed on the Binet visual test, already mentioned, and could not name the months in order, but, on the other hand, three of the fifteen-year tests were well done. Where common sense or reasoning was required, responses were correct and quite prompt. Absurdities were detected, and even the fifteen-year tests for interpretation and inference caused him no trouble.

The boy was poorly informed, possibly due to the fact that he read very little. Indeed, we soon found that he was unable to read a third-grade passage with any degree of fluency or accuracy. He often failed on even simple words, substituting some word that the context suggested. Having stumbled slowly through a passage he could reproduce the meaning. His difficulty lay in recognition of the symbols. Many words had to be sounded first phonetically. Spelling was similarly poor: he wrote, "The prenter mad some cors." In number work he was inaccurate in carrying out the processes, although he understood the principles involved and knew the number combinations. He very rapidly gave the multiplication tables orally, making only one error when he said "ten times twelve is one hundred and two." Perhaps it would be stretching the point to interpret this error as certainly due to a wrong visual picture, but this interpretation is interesting at least as a possibility. Reasoning powers, as shown on simple arithmetical problems as well as in a number of other tests, seemed quite normal.

We have here, then, a boy who shows a decided difference in auditory and visual powers, the former being distinctly good and the latter decidedly below normal. So far as he was tested, anything in the auditory field was done extremely well.

Physically the boy was fairly well developed, but rather poorly nourished. There may have been some difficulty with adenoids, for he was a partial mouth-breather. He had suffered no illnesses, except that when he was seven years old he had fallen, striking the back of his head, and two weeks later went to the hospital because paralysis of the left side then appeared. He was said to have been unable to talk for about ten days, but then recovered his speech. At the time of our examination, we found no speech defect of any kind. Evidently he made a good recovery; when we saw him there was but very slight atrophy of the left side, knee jerks were almost equal, and there was very little difference noted in the strength of the two arms; he walked with a slight limp.

Case 25. Edgar M., 11 years old, has had the best of opportunities, both from the standpoint of home environment and continuous attendance at an unusually fine school. Every advantage that comes from intelligent home interest and coöperation has been his. By his regular teachers and occasional tutors much effort has been expended in the desire to help the boy progress. In spite of all this, he was brought to us by his highly intelligent parents as a case which was perhaps not understood and which was felt to be met unsatisfactorily by the ordinary school procedure. He was not a disciplinary problem, but he showed extremely little interest in school work, and little initiative or response even in outside activities. His range of interests was said to be very limited.

Our several psychological examinations revealed the fact that in many respects Edgar was far beyond his age in ability, in spite of his poor standing in school. As judged by the Binet scale, his general intelligence was much in advance of his chronological age, for he passed all the tests through the twelve and fifteen-year groups readily. His apperceptions were exceedingly keen and good, as was shown in many ways. Not only did he do well on psychological tests for apperception, but he showed an unusually keen sense of humor for a boy of his age, very quickly perceiving the point of a joke or riddle, and his social apperceptions, as shown by his good manners and general politeness, corroborated the findings on tests. Then, too, his reasoning ability we discovered to be far beyond the norm for his age. This was evidenced by a variety of tests in this field, including such fairly difficult tasks as the analogies test designed for fifteen-year old children. He very quickly perceived the relationships involved and made not a single error in any test of this kind.

Tests requiring a number of abilities, as in the difficult directions test, were done extremely well, with good powers of attention and concentration, with full appreciation of the "catches", and with a very rational understanding of all that was required. Processes of association as tested in several ways were normal. These included both free and controlled verbal associations and the formation of new associations between arbitrary symbols, in which the boy showed quite good learning ability. Tests for analysis and mental representation were done correctly too, but in the more difficult of these it was apparent that the visual powers were not any aid, and the solution was largely by means of reasoning out the situations. As for memory, there was found a distinct difference in the auditory and visual fields, the former being considerably better. This was true both for rote and logical material. Whereas the boy could remember readily eight numerals heard once, it was extraordinary to note that he had difficulty in remembering seven presented visually, and succeeded then only by translating visual into auditory terms. A passage read to him was reproduced very well, only one item out of twelve being omitted, but when he himself read a passage, the reproduction was considerably worse, only thirteen out of twenty items being recalled.

In connection with his poor visual memory, it was interesting to observe that all visual perceptions were extremely slow. In the construction test, where the problems require the perception of relationships of form, the procedure was rational, but very slow. Again in the apperception test the boy very quickly gave the meaning of the situations depicted pictorially, but was very slow in finding the pieces he wished to insert, showing that his apperceptions were quicker than his visual perceptions.

This slowness of perception and innate lack of good visual power was strikingly apparent on the so-called Aussage test, where after seeing a picture for a brief time an account of it is given, after which questions are asked concerning points not voluntarily mentioned. In this test the boy distinctly showed his disability; he gave only five items in the free account and was exceedingly uncertain in regard to other points about which he was questioned. He often said, "I don't know", or "I'm not sure", and some of the more prominent objects depicted were not seen by him at all. His performance here was very much worse than that of many a child who is actually younger, to say nothing of less generally intelligent than he. Coupled with his slowness in visual perception, there was quite a little difficulty in motor coördination. He was unable to make a good record on the so-called tapping test, and his poor writing indicated, too, this lack of psychomotor control.

In school the difficulty had partly been to arouse and

maintain the boy's interest. He was retarded in arithmetic; he had learned to add, subtract, and to multiply, all of which he did slowly; in long division, however, he was exceedingly inaccurate. He failed on several simple examples given him. In spite of his very good reasoning powers he did not do well in arithmetical problems. He read fluently and as well as could be expected for his age and grade. He gave a good reproduction of the ideas contained in the passage, but even so he much preferred being read to; he himself said, "I am too lazy to read it", and the physical side of the process seemed irksome. Another school question arose from the fact that he wrote so slowly and so poorly, in consequence of which his spelling was not up to the standard of his class.

The peculiarities in Edgar's mental make-up revealed by the psychological tests become significant for understanding the school record which so puzzled his teachers and parents. His difficulty in visual perception and his slowness in this field had been a very great handicap in many of the schoolroom activities. He could not perceive at a normal rate such work as was put upon the blackboard, or even what he read from books. Certainly, however, his perception of ideas was normal. It is only through meeting such a problem that we realize how much of school work requires normal powers of visual perception.

The poor visual memory which this boy demonstrated undoubtedly also entered into the situation, but since he transposes so readily visual into auditory terms, this probably was not so great a factor as his other difficulty, namely, poor motor coördinations. Slowness in visual perceptions and slowness in writing due to his poor motor coördinations explain his retardation in spite of his very unusual abilities in so many ways. In oral recitations where reasoning is involved, or where general intelligence or ability to grasp meaning is the main element, this boy would do extremely well, but since a large part of the ordinary schoolroom procedure deals with mechanical elements difficult for him, he is at a great disadvantage.

Other facts regarding the boy are as follows: Edgar was born in England, but came with his parents to this country when a very small lad and began school at the usual age, attending regularly. The heredity and developmental history are entirely negative. Physically he is decidedly small for his age, but quite well nourished. His considerable myopia has been corrected by glasses since he was six years old. No other sensory defects have been noted in the course of examinations by the best of specialists. He seemed rather lacking in energy and vigor. Physical reactions have all his life been notably quiet, though he is a healthy boy.

On the constructive side, concerning what could be done in such a case, one naturally thinks of several possible plans. With individual help perhaps much might be accomplished through systematic training to improve his powers of visual perception. All kinds of devices could be employed to give practice in the visual field, so that his perceptions would become more rapid. The same is true regarding psychomotor control. Corrective gymnastics and games, first simple and then becoming more and more difficult, ought to be a great help to him. And then much school work which now stresses, or indeed taxes, the perceptual side, could be eliminated in favor of other methods of presentation. Thorndike has made the point that no work in the schoolroom is as trying on the eyes as the copying of numbers from the blackboard, and has suggested that much eye strain could be saved by giving arithmetic work in books where the problems are already written and only the solution need be set down.   There is a tremendous waste of time, effort, and nervous energy in the amount of copying that is demanded of children in the ordinary schoolroom without any profit accruing from the task.   All children suffer thereby, and in a case such as the one under discussion the penalty is extreme.

In the case of Edgar several matters pertaining to the physical side of his make-up were taken into serious consideration.   In the first place, thinking of the basis of his defects, what part did his myopia play in possibly preventing the acquisition of ordinary visual impressions and perceptions, in preventing the mind from being stored to anything like the normal extent with visual imagery? Easy though it may be to suggest such causation, it is quite impossible to affirm that myopia was or could have been the main factor.   It is true that up to his sixth year Edgar was gaining but poor impressions of the seen world, but during the succeeding five years eyesight was nearly normal.   Besides, plenty of other children who have suffered as much early in life from myopia have not later shown such marked disability for visual perceptions.   And why should the visual difficulty have affected visual memory to the extent of creating a defect? All together, it seems to us, the probability is that the origin of the defect in this case lies much deeper than early imperfect vision.

Then, the question whether the general physical condition was responsible for lack of interest and initiative was considered.   The only way to answer this was to observe the effects of appropriate physical treatment.   There was no problem of general health, — Edgar was quite up to the average in this respect, — but he had not grown normally, so far; he was decidedly small for his age.   And the remarkable quietness of his physical reactions, we felt, might portend that the sources of physical energy were not well maintained. He had suffered from recurrent adenoids, but these, as well as any other slight ailment, were promptly cared for under the best of advice. We thought of general physiological problems of metabolism and their relation to internal gland secretions. With a view to improving any fault of this kind, if it existed, appropriate treatment was instituted.

At this time our findings were presented to Edgar's teachers in conference and they, appreciating thoroughly his problem, began anew, now with different methods, to coöperate with the parents in stimulating and instructing him. Some have suggested that the bare fact of a study having been made of his case and new interest taken in him, has led Edgar to become more conscious of his difficulties and has really awakened him to better efforts, which of themselves have largely turned the tide.

As in many instances where a satisfactory treatment has been introduced, the relative values of the several changes are hard to determine. At any rate, the results in this case have been most gratifying. While no essential physical changes were observed, Edgar began very soon to show new interest in his work, to make unprecedented headway, and to maintain well his standing in his class. It is reported that in the year which has elapsed since we first saw him, he has shown great advance in mental energy and in acquisitions.

DISABILITIES FOR WORK WITH CONCRETE MATERIAL

In considering ability and disability for manual work, we must again remember that distinctions exist between activities that may seem on the surface much alike. It is one thing to be unable to solve problems dealing with concrete material because of difficulty in finding methods of solution, and quite a different thing to produce a poor result because of lack of dexterity to carry out well the solution one has reached. The former depends upon ability to reason regarding situations involving perception of concrete relationships. Ruger [1] has shown the individual differences that exist in ability to solve puzzles, where methods employed by intelligent college-trained subjects vary all the way from random trial and error to deliberated planfulness, based on analysis and reasoning.

Acquisition of manual skill necessary to carry ideas into execution depends on good psychomotor control and effective coördinations. Where there is disability in psychomotor control, perception of relationship may be normal, the method of solution quickly seen, but the ability to carry out the plan of procedure is poor, because the neural connections leading to movement are faulty.

There has been some recognition of differences in ability to perform manual work, though the emphasis has been placed more often on unusual ability in this direction in individuals who are generally dull or unable to progress normally in work dealing with abstractions. Holmes [2] speaks of individuals with "concrete minds" or "manual minds." On the other hand, very frequently too little cognizance is taken of defects for dealing with concrete problems. Perhaps it is therefore wise to stress the fact that disabilities of this kind exist. More and more handwork is being offered in schools, and it seems quite generally taken for granted that all children are fitted for this type of work. While we do not doubt that some benefit is to be derived from such training, even by those not possessed of manual skill, yet the general educational and vocational aspects are extremely important to keep in mind.

[1] Ruger, A. H., "Psychology of Efficiency." *Archives of Psychology*, 15.

[2] Holmes, Arthur. "The Backward Child." 1915.

From among a number of instances that we have met, an illustration of educational and vocational misplacing made because of lack of appreciation of this type of defect is cited.

Case 26. Melvin W., 15 years old, was American born, of foreign parentage. He had attended public school from his sixth year, but had been such an extreme truant that three times he had been committed to a school for such offenders. Both there and at another correctional institution where he was held for some time the main emphasis is placed on manual training, although the usual school subjects are also taught.

The findings on psychological tests in this case were very striking because of the discrepancy between results on tests for constructive ability, as shown in the handling of concrete material, and on those involving abstractions. We must take into consideration the unusual amount of training along motor lines which Melvin had received. In spite of the months spent in shop work, the boy could not perform well any test with concrete material that required perception of relationships or needed any independent thinking or judgment. He had learned to do certain simple tasks through imitation; given the parts which were to make an object, the model of which was before him, he succeeded; that is, he could copy from the model the steps required, but where the purpose was stated and he himself had to find the method to achieve the end, he was a dismal failure. Simple construction tests frequently done by normal eight-year-old children proved too difficult for him. He solved them only by random methods, showing not the slightest comprehension of the problems as such; he did not profit by his own mistakes, but kept repeating them, with slight apperceptions in the face of this kind of situation. He was extremely awkward in the use of his hands, demonstrating decidedly poor psychomotor control. He seemed quite unable to size up any practical, concrete situation, even such as Terman's Ball and Field Puzzle, where the person is asked to tell the best method that can be used in finding a ball lost in a circular field of high grass. In the Yerkes Multiple Choice test, which so specially tests ability to form generalizations on the basis of repeated experience with concrete situations, his record on the first two problems was considerably worse than the tentative norms for untrained subjects.   Indeed, a variety of tests, all requiring the same kind of ability, namely, judgment or skill with actual material, corroborated each other.

But on work of different types the boy did quite well. Tests for the powers of mental analysis and mental representation caused him no trouble, and he showed normal apperceptions of ideas expressed verbally. He was able to do normally the so-called directions test. His verbal associations were normal, and we found no trouble with memory in any phase. In repeating the ideas contained in a logical passage, he was hampered by poor knowledge of English, yet the main ideas themselves were reproduced. In the substitution learning test he made a good record, and reasoning powers required for response to common-sense questions, in the detection of incongruities and in arithmetical problems, were quite good.

Of routine school work Melvin had not acquired a great deal, but we felt that there was no defect for work of this type, since one had to take into consideration the excessive truancy which had been a feature of his entire school life. When we first saw him he was inaccurate in all work in arithmetic, although he knew the processes and number combinations. At that time he read only haltingly, mispronouncing less commonly met words, but he could give the gist of what he read. Our explanation of these rather poor results proved to be correct, for with three months' training in these school branches he gained vastly. When the same work was tried at the expiration of this time, we found that he had learned to add, subtract, multiply, and divide correctly and quickly. He had improved quite a little in his writing and spelling, and somewhat in reading, though this was still not very good.

He came from a rather poor home; both father and mother were dull, hard-working people. They lived in a congested neighborhood where the boy was thrown with bad companions. Indeed, Melvin had been in court repeatedly over a period of two years, involved in truancy, stealing, and burglary with the same group of boys. The problem was that of a typical street gang, and neither the home nor the neighborhood offered anything to substitute for the misconduct that characterized these boys. We were unable to obtain from the dull parents any facts of significance in regard to the heredity, but we noted in the physical examination of the boy evidences of congenital lues; a blood test, however, resulted in a negative reaction. Neither were we able to obtain a good developmental history. Our physical examination showed that there were no sensory defects nor any signs of nervous disturbance. The boy was fairly well developed, and himself said that he had never been very ill.

Concerning education, this case illustrates the fallacy of a very common procedure. It seems to be quite a prevalent idea that the main training undertaken in correctional institutions ought to be along the lines of manual work. Of course numerous considerations enter in, and for boys of a certain age no doubt trade training is to be advocated in order that upon release they may be fitted for an occupation which will make them economically successful. But there are some, like Melvin, who are incapable of profiting much by the expenditure of this educational effort and who would, perhaps, succeed far better in work which would prepare them, let us say, for employment in an office. Our diagnosis in regard to this boy's lack of ability for manual tasks was in accord with the reports given us by his manual training teachers. One of them said in regard to Melvin that the boy had to be shown what to do step by step, and then the instructor had to stand over him to see that he did it. Although he had been given a considerable amount of individual help, he was unable to carry out any planning by himself. He showed no initiative or originality in the work, no ability to use material in a rational way. The teacher himself felt confident that the boy would never be successful at this type of work.

With his inadequate school training because of his excessive truancy, the boy really was unfitted for any employment. He had previously been placed at jobs that were along the line of his greatest incapacity. He worked in factories and had not been successful. Once he had been placed, through his probation officer, in a carpenter shop. We can easily see what should have been done in this case. Instead of the time devoted to shop work, the boy should have had intensive training in writing and number work, or something of a type which would have made it possible for him to succeed at clerical work, or at least in some position where he would not have had to do skilled manual work.

Case 27. A record can be given of a few tests which show extreme difficulty in solving problems with concrete material, unaccompanied by poor psychomotor control, and in great contrast to results on other types of tests.

Alexander T., 13 years and 9 months of age, was a serious boy who made great efforts to do well all that was asked of him. He worked persistently and with good powers of attention. In spite of his earnest endeavors, the results on tests with concrete material were uniformly poor. The simpler construction test, solved usually by young children, he did by a purely random method, numerous impossibilities being repeated again and again. Perception of relationships was no better on the more difficult construction test; here the boy seemed utterly unable to work in any rational way. He tried every possible combination, repeating his errors, and finally at the end of five minutes had not succeeded. On the Stenquist test for mechanical ability, he demonstrated no more skill; he worked persistently, but at the end of a half hour he had not completed all of the models. The simpler models were correctly copied, but the lock was not put together properly, several of the parts being omitted, a fact which Alexander did not appreciate. One of the simplest models was not correctly bolted together; the placing of a single rubber band over pegs to form a five-pointed star caused the greatest trouble. Although the boy looked at the copy most carefully and persisted for twenty-three minutes in his efforts to place the rubber band, he finally gave it up.

No awkwardness whatever was displayed in his manipulation of concrete material, and tests gave no evidence of any difficulty in psychomotor control. On both the tapping test and the instructions box he made a good record. His writing of words and figures was rapid and remarkably neat.

On tests of other types responses were prompt and normal. Both cross-line tests were solved correctly on first trial. Apperceptions, as shown on the completion test, were rapid and accurate. School work was done well for his grade, and according to the Binet scale the boy graded as normal. His delinquencies were no doubt due to factors other than his special disability; the latter doubtless would play a great rôle later in vocational life.

DEFECT IN SPEED OF REACTIONS

In any study of performance there are two factors which need to be considered. On the one hand, there is the accuracy of the reaction ; on the other hand, there is the speed of the reaction. In evaluating test results, both factors, accuracy and speed, are frequently combined. In different kinds of work either the one or the other may be the more important factor of the two.

Though both in school and later in the business world the emphasis shifts back and forth from one to the other, now speed, now accuracy being more important, at no time is either altogether negligible. The problem in arithmetic, for example, must be solved correctly, but also rapidly enough to be completed within certain limits of time. The child who cannot keep up with the average of the class because of slowness of mental reactions is at a very great disadvantage. Even though he understands his work and can perform it correctly if given long enough time, he becomes an out-and-out school failure if unable to complete tasks as promptly as is required. In industrial life speed is often a very vital consideration.

Many experimental studies of reaction types have been made, and though the explanation of differences in speed may be obscure, inasmuch as we do not know whether all or only part of the active neural mechanism is at fault, the fact that there is great variability in reaction time is well known. Slowness of reaction leads to practical consequences even early in life. Holmes [1] cites an interesting case of a child who because of his general slowness was most unfortunately considered a dunce in school, but who later when properly adjusted vocationally was a tremendous success. Almost everyone is acquainted with people who are intelligent enough, but who are slow.

[1] Holmes, Arthur. "The Backward Child." 1915,

Sometimes this inability to react quickly is characteristic of all responses, and sometimes it is true only in special fields.

That slowness of mental reactions is sometimes the explanation of seeming general incapacity is illustrated by the following case:

Case 28. Arthur R., 17 years old, was a boy who had exceedingly good educational advantages, but he was considered by his family and his teachers, and so ultimately by himself, to be a failure. Because of his poor school record and his general slowness, his quick-minded family categorized him as innately stupid, and now, at this late age, desired a study made of his difficulties and educational possibilities.

Mental tests given to this young man showed a significant difference from normal achievement, not so much because of inability to succeed with the problems and tasks, but because of the unusually long time the performance nearly always required. This characteristic was even evident when Arthur was working with concrete material, though less so than with abstract; perceptions of form and of relationships of form were accurate but slow. In problems dealing with the concrete he learned fairly readily and retained what he learned. His apperceptions, though normal, were exceedingly slow; his record on the pictorial completion test indicates that he required at least twice the amount of time that is ordinarily needed by a normal person of Arthur's age. When the task was completed, however, no errors were made. It was interesting to compare results on memory tests for logical material with memory span and to interpret the distinct difference that was found. On the former far better results were achieved than on the latter. On tests for logical material, the reproduction does not follow as quickly as in tests for memory span. The subject reads the passage as slowly as he wishes when presentation is visual, and when it is auditory the passage is read to him several times. But, in testing the memory span the reproduction is immediate, the numbers being read but once and the visual stimulus exposed but ten seconds.

Given sufficient time, Arthur showed normal ability to analyze and reason, but in all tests where time is considered significant, the results were distinctly poor. On the very easy substitution test, two errors were made on the first trial and none on the second, indicating the exceeding slowness with which associations of arbitrary symbols were formed. The Kraepelin test was performed without error, but very slowly and deliberately. In the attempt to open the puzzle box, the boy studied the situation for five minutes before making the first move, after which the task was completed very rapidly. Some tests which he failed to solve in the laboratory he worked out by pondering over them until the examination of the next day. Tests requiring the use of language revealed also Arthur's characteristic slowness of mental reaction. All were ultimately correct, but he was slow both in comprehending a situation presented verbally and in expressing his own ideas. It was quite surprising to find that this boy of good education and coming from a home of culture should have much trouble in forming a sentence containing three assigned words or in stating clearly distinctions between a king and a president. In school work he did very poorly, especially arithmetic, where even addition, though done correctly, took a very great deal of time. Errors were made in multiplication and division.

If the performances are carefully analyzed, it is found that this boy is not lacking in any of the higher thought processes. He shows good powers of analysis and mental representation, reasoning, planfulness, and fairly good mental control. The extreme slowness with which the mental processes function is the most striking feature of all his work. His inability to use language well, to express his own ideas in clear and forceful form, probably is due to his inability to formulate his ideas quickly. Perhaps if his answers had been written and he had been able to revise them, taking as much time as he desired, as in the case of the problems he solved overnight, he might have been able to prove that he has good ability in this direction too.

He was said to have walked and talked at a much later age than other members of the family; developmental history in other ways was entirely negative. Not until a year previously was it known that the boy had defective vision in one eye. As for his education, he had been sent to the very best of private schools; he had been tried three times in the public schools, but was always unable to succeed there. The boy himself said that he liked arithmetic pretty well, but could never succeed in it, and that he "never was any good" in history or grammar.

No doubt this boy would be at great disadvantage everywhere in the ordinary classroom when competing with students who have no special disabilities. Defective vision could hardly have been the important factor, for such tests as the association and other language tests would not have been affected thereby. If he required much more time to perform mental operations than the average child, of course he would naturally be regarded as quite unable to do many things on which he failed, not through lack of real capacity, but because of the insufficient time allowed him.

Whether much might have been done to stimulate this boy and train him so that he could think more quickly is an interesting question, but one we cannot answer. We are sure that the ordinary schoolroom emphasizes the time of the reactions as well as accuracy, and this is, doubtless, as it should be. Where, however, there is a particular lack of ability to react promptly, what can be done to improve the situation? Ought a person of whom this slowness is characteristic to be taught under the same conditions that succeed with the ordinary child? If no allowance is made for the mental peculiarity, can one expect the child to develop without discouragements that must impede his progress all the more? It is evident that retardation under ordinary school methods is inevitable. The results of falling back would be likely to be much more serious in producing depression and discouragement in the case of a person really normal than would be true if there were general mental defect. Sensibilities and emotions being as in the ordinary individual, consequences might be disastrous indeed.

In the case of Arthur we felt that it was sound advice to suggest that he be trained for an occupation that requires no swift reactions. Some types of manufacturing or of laboratory work, or, still better, agriculture in any one of its diverse forms, would be suitable as a life work. In some such pursuit his really good intelligence would be likely to lead to success.

DEFECTS IN PERCEPTUAL ABILITIES

Individual differences in sensory and perceptual powers are clearly shown by many experiments with various problems in these fields. Discrimination of weight, color, form, length of line, etc., have been studied, as well as many other types of tactile, visual, auditory, and other perceptions. Capacity in these processes, from whatever standpoint they are considered, varies greatly. Disability extreme enough to be denominated a defect refers in this discussion, of course, to conditions that do not rest on the basis of defective sensory organs, but are due to some lack of functioning in the central nervous system.

From the practical standpoint such defects are of vital significance in relation to the activities of everyday life, where perceptual discriminations of all sorts are constantly demanded. But the fact is that in spite of much experimentation we do not know the thresholds below which disability in perceptual powers, auditory, visual, or for stimuli of other types, becomes important as conditioning failure in educational and vocational life. The correlation between such defects, more or less extreme, and mental activities, such as the school subjects and industrial occupations represent, have been, as yet, little studied and are almost undetermined. But that such defective powers lie at the root of some school and vocational failures we have learned from experience.

Only the following case-history is cited, because defects in visual and auditory perceptions have been dealt with under other headings; this case presents disability in other perceptions.

Case 29. Agnes Z., 8 years old, was brought from an eastern city for study because it had already been found that she could not be taught by ordinary methods. She had been tried in the public schools, but without success, and her parents very wisely recognized that in order to succeed with her, they ought to know her problem and learn the best methods of coping with it.

In spite of the reported difficulty in learning, we found on psychological examination that this girl could not be regarded as an out-and-out mental defective; by the Binet scale she was just one year retarded, but this meant little that was helpful in understanding her mental make-up. The interesting fact revealed by Binet and even more clearly by other tests was the unevenness of abilities, for some things were done extremely well and others equally as poorly. Young as she was, certain results on tests gave clues that could be seen to be most important from the standpoint of her further education.

Sensory discrimination and perceptions were very good as related to color, but extremely poor for form and relationships of form. Whereas she readily distinguished the colors and combined the pieces of a picture puzzle test when the picture was a colored one, she had great difficulty in doing an analogous task when not assisted by the element of color; that is, when she had to rely upon form. She was unable to solve even the simpler of the construction tests, and she was quite unsuccessful in remembering the solution; she learned to put the pieces properly into place only after she had been shown how to do so repeatedly. Perceptions of weight were very faulty too; she could not select the heavier of two weights, one weighing three, the other twelve grams.

Although memory for form relationships was so notably poor, she had an unusually good rote memory for verbal material. She memorized poems rapidly, having, however, a great deal of difficulty in giving the meaning of the selection. She had learned in the same way number combinations, but had not the slightest concept of number. She could add a series of digits, but could not perform the same steps with stamps or money, nor reason on the basis of the number combinations which she knew. Her memory for language was far better than her ability to use language as a medium of expression. In the one case she was rather above her age, as determined by psychological tests, and in the others she was quite below the standard for her age.

Her powers of apperception were unusually good. She showed quite good common sense for her years, readily grasped the situations presented in various tests, and showed normal appreciations of what constitutes good social behavior. She interpreted pictures well, showing here, too, normal perceptions of colors and objects. As for other disabilities, we found that she had much trouble with psychomotor control, as indicated by tests and by her great difficulty with the writing of letters and numbers.

The results of the training in school work which she had received were exceedingly interesting. She could read fluently, but had some little difficulty in giving the meaning of what she read. She could spell quite well, but her writing, as above mentioned, was quite illegible. She had acquired quite a little general information and much in the way of poetry, which she recited, however, in parrot-like fashion. She could add correctly, but even this had no real meaning for her. No doubt she would not have learned as much as this except for the very good individual instruction which was being given her. For about a year she had been under the direction of a special teacher, but the latter had not undertaken to make any definite diagnosis of mentality, basing work merely on experience with what was and what was not successful.

The practical problem in this case was to determine the educational possibilities and the methods to be employed. It will be readily understood that Agnes needed a great deal of training in form perception, which probably she could obtain less well by working with flat surfaces than with solid objects. We advised that she learn to use a scroll-saw and develop her perception of form by putting together parts of pictures which she herself had cut out. Appreciation of form relationships needed developing, which could well be done through various games. In connection with this, there would naturally come some special training in motor control. Perhaps even her writing would be more improved by general training for psychomotor control than by practice in that particular activity. Many devices, of course, could be employed for this purpose. Then, too, she needed to be trained to use language as a medium for the expression of her own ideas. For this there are numerous devices which would give her practice. The ability to perceive rational relationships and logical connection between things would no doubt develop with more training and experience and with increasing maturity of mental powers.

In her school work it is the meaning of what is read that should be emphasized, and the number concepts brought out that lie back of addition and subtraction and the other processes of arithmetic. Rote memory, in which she excels, would, of course, be called into play constantly, the danger being that she would rely upon it too much. It is just such powers that often obscure the fact that ideas are not really mastered. By stressing the rational phases of activities and leading her to acquire an interest in them, no doubt she would develop more initiative in regard to work, both in school and out of it. Of course, this little girl's naturally good powers in certain directions should also be utilized, but they are, in general, of such a character that they would always be bound to come into play, whereas her disabilities might be unrealized simply because facility on the basis of memory would carry her along quite well for many purposes. To know just wherein this girl is lacking and where she needs particular help and training ought to mean much for the success of her education. Naturally, the putting of such advice into practice requires an intelligent and well-trained teacher, one who can appreciate the psychological aspects of the case, and who has skill and ingenuity in devising means for applying the principles involved.

From the intelligent mother we obtained a very good account of heredity and developmental conditions. The former was entirely negative. There had been some antenatal difficulty, the mother not being well during the pregnancy. Agnes weighed only three and one half pounds at birth and for a long time afterwards was badly nourished. At six months she weighed only four or five pounds, but by the time she was a year old, nourishing food had been found, and she became quite normal in weight. She suffered from numerous illnesses; at six weeks she had a severe attack of pneumonia, at four years she was very ill with measles, and at six years had typhoid fever, but made a very good recovery. She did not walk or talk until three years old. Dentition was late. We found her, at eight years old, physically normal in general development, and all examination was negative except that she had defective vision which was corrected by glasses.

DEFECTS IN THE HIGHER MENTAL PROCESSES

Defects in the higher mental processes must be discussed, although the presence of such defects leads one to doubt whether the individual possessing them can be regarded as sufficiently normal mentally to fall within the group belonging to our discussion, namely, normal individuals with special defect. Powers of apperception, reasoning, judgment, mental representation, and foresight, are naturally criteria of intelligence to such an extent that defects in these aspects of mental life would seem to indicate subnormality, if not feeble-mindedness. But as a matter of fact, there are individuals who lack some one of these mental powers, yet who do well in many other tasks not involving the defect. Frequently there is great difficulty in deciding whether such an individual is normal or subnormal; many are ultimately designated as "border-line." Of course, as we have already stated, it must be carefully realized that apperceptions or reasoning power or judgment may be faulty in specialized fields, owing to lack of experience which would give the individual the data necessary to perform these mental functions.

Sometimes, however, a person proves that he has normal capacity as judged by his social reactions or by the results on ordinary mental tests, and yet he may have extremely poor ability in some one or more of the so-called higher mental powers, even in relation to situations with which he is familiar. He may not be keen in reasoning, or his judgment may not be good, or he may act without prudence and foresight. It is true that extreme disability in apperception is often an indication of aberrational tendencies, but even normal individuals vary greatly in their capacity for sizing up situations.

While we cannot here cover this topic of our problem thoroughly, we cite several cases illustrating defects in higher mental powers. Whether the individuals can be classified as of normal intelligence may sometimes be open to question, but though they have such clearly seen defects, they likewise have such striking abilities in many other fields that they are more properly placed in this chapter than in the later one devoted to subnormal individuals with special abilities.

Mental representation: In the case given below, very poor results were attained on many tasks, results which we believe may be explained by extreme disability in powers of mental representation. Discussing the place of this mental trait, Healy says, "The ability to represent in terms of various imageries a given situation to oneself, and to revolve it over in the mind, seeing its different parts, and mentally commenting on their comparisons and relationships, is one of the most valuable of human faculties." [1]

Case 30. The defective power of mental representation is here coupled with great lack in visual imagery.

Leonard B., 17 years, 11 months old, was brought us for study by his mother, a very intelligent woman, because he was not succeeding in school work. He had been attending school since six years old. He had had tutors at various times, some of them very good teachers, "but they never made anything of him." In spite of having had private instruction for an entire year, in the hope of preparing him for high school, the boy was not able to maintain his position in the seventh grade. He was not a delinquent, but his family had supplied him with many wholesome interests which had done much to prevent a growth of harmful tendencies.

The psychological examination presented a most complex problem, for the results in general were exceedingly irregular, many tests being done very well, and others, readily performed by much younger children, were in some instances poorly done and in others complete failures. The problem here becomes one for analysis. We must try to find, if possible, what mental processes are involved in the successes and failures in order to determine if they throw any light on the boy's inability to progress at school.

Analysis of successful records shows that Leonard did very well on tests with concrete material, that his perceptions of form and form relationships were normal, or above. He succeeded on construction tests, working promptly and understandingly. Once such problems were solved, he gained by his own experience; he performed them the second time much more rapidly, showing

[1] Healy, William. "The Individual Delinquent." 1914.

that he had grasped the principles involved and that he remembered them. He showed, too, ability to reason concerning any problems thus presented, solving them by rational, planful methods. Psychomotor control was likewise good; in all phases of manual work he had unusually good ability. By Binet tests he graded as normal, and on school work he had no difficulty with reading and writing. He talked well concerning things in which he was interested and had distinctly good apperceptions, both as required on tests and regarding his own disabilities.

The tests on which he failed seemed on the surface to be quite unlike each other. They were those to test powers of mental analysis and mental representation, ability to form new associations between arbitrary symbols, ability to follow directions after the experimenter has shown the steps of the process, as in the instructions box. Results on tests for memory indicated variability in the different aspects; rote memory for auditory presentations was normal, auditory memory for logical material could scarcely be considered either exceptionally good or poor; about two thirds of the passage was recalled. But visual memory was astonishingly poor. The boy could not draw from memory a simple figure seen over and over again, nor could he make a recognizable representation of so simple an object as an ink bottle. Having been shown the figure used in the cross line test, consisting of two parallel vertical lines and two parallel horizontal lines, he could not draw the figure correctly. In the adult Binet tests where mental representation is required, as for example in reconstructing the triangles, Leonard failed completely. Almost all work in arithmetic was quite beyond his ability. He could add and subtract correctly, but he could neither multiply nor divide; and the addition of fractions was a complete failure. More striking still was the fact that in very simple problems he could state the reasoning required in the solution, but could not carry out the process. Thus, given such an example as, If one dozen apples cost fifty-four cents, how much will eight apples cost? he quickly said, "You must find the cost of one and then get eight times that amount," yet he could not give the answer. In continuous subtraction, taking seven from one hundred orally, he made six errors. On other school work it was found that his spelling was poor and his knowledge of geography slight.

Comparing now the failures and successes, we are at once impressed by the contrast presented. Inability to handle the abstract as compared with his successful achievements with concrete material is striking. In an effort to explain the poor records made on various tests, let us analyze still further the functions required. Is one justified in concluding that the great lack, as seen in the case of this boy, is the power of mental representation? It would seem as though his failure in tasks apparently very different might indicate a lack of ability to represent to himself mentally, either in visual or other form, the successive steps in a process. His inability to follow directions when six or seven steps are demanded, and his failure on such a test as that for continuous subtraction, might both be due to a lack of ability in mental representation. There is, too, obvious defect in visual memory which may be a large feature in his inability to represent to himself the task in hand, particularly when the transformation into terms other than visual is difficult. This might account for his failure in spelling, where he shows difficulty in mental representation of words which had been presented to him probably in their visual form, and his inaccuracy in geography could be accounted for in the same way. The latter, we note, was never presented to him except by the usual methods, that is, by the use of flat maps interpreted largely in visual terms and appealing to memory through visual representation.

No facts of significance regarding heredity were obtained from the intelligent mother, whose account, no doubt, was altogether reliable. Developmental history was negative. There were only mild illnesses, and no physical disabilities of any kind were noted at the time of our examination.

Considering Leonard's distinct disability for handling abstractions and his equally distinct ability in working with concrete material, it seems reasonable to infer that the methods of instruction which had been employed in his case had not been adapted to his mental make-up. His training should have been largely along manual lines. No doubt he might have succeeded well in any of the practical applied sciences which involve the use of machinery or other kind of apparatus. Even the ordinary school work might have been mastered with a far greater degree of success had the presentations been through concrete means. Indeed, we are sure of this from the results of teaching geography to Leonard for a couple of months along the lines we prescribed. He acquired "more than he had learned in his whole life before."

Perceptions of relationship: Some psychologists have included in their enumeration of the various mental processes the group of functions designated as feelings or perceptions of relationship. In general we may distinguish between objective relationships, such as those of space and form, and subjective relationships, such as likeness, equality, cause and effect, and other logical relations. It is quite possible that defects may exist in either one or the other and even in both these subdivisions. If there can be specialized defect for time sense, as seems likely from the peculiarities noted in cases of aberration where time orientation is often exceedingly poor, for instance, in Korsakow's syndrome, we should say that it is a specialized defect in the realm of perception of objective relationships. The same conclusion would be true in regard to a possibly defective sense of form. In contradistinction, defects concerning subjective relationships would affect reasoning, and, indeed, all logical thinking.

Case 31. In the following case is seen defect for perceptions of relationship, both objective and subjective; we find here inability to perceive relationships as they exist in both concrete and abstract problems.

Julian M., 14 years of age, often a truant and a great mischief maker in school, was studied on the mental side with much care, because of the great irregularities that were found in the results on different tests. The boy's educational advantages had been good. He had been in several public schools and more recently in an expensive private school, known for its thoroughness and successful achievements.

Judged by general intelligence tests the boy graded as normal; he passed through the twelve-year Binet tests without any failures. In school subjects he was up to grade in reading, writing, and spelling. No unusual features were detected in any of these subjects. He did well on the test for learning ability as evidenced in forming associations between arbitrary symbols. Memory processes were normal, both for rote and logical material. He was able to follow directions, making quite a good record on special tests for this, nor had he any difficulty with tests for analysis and mental representation where the relationships were explicitly shown him.

On the other hand, he failed badly on all other tests requiring perceptions of relationship, either in abstractions or in the concrete. He showed poor powers of reasoning and little foresight when the latter was a factor in tests, and his apperceptive ability, as gauged in the laboratory, was notably poor for a boy of his age. He did not succeed in solving the simplest puzzles which require recognition of relationships of form. On tests presented in concrete form he used purely random methods. Thus, in the opening of the so-called puzzle box his record was extremely poor; he studied the box a long time, quite unable to plan any mode of procedure, finally adopting a method that was purely trial and error. Indeed, he made many errors which reason or even quick perception would have made impossible. On the pictorial completion test the errors made were significant not only because of their number, but even more because of their type. He showed great lack of ability to select pieces which bore sensible relationships to the incidents depicted in this test. He played a poor game of checkers, taking no advantage of obvious chances, although he maintained he had played this game frequently. He did not grasp the principle of the code test until elaborate explanations were given, after which he was able to cope with the test fairly well. Not only was he poorly informed, but events were poorly placed and quite unrelated in time. Thus, he informed us that the fourth of July was celebrated as Washington's birthday; that Lincoln, who was a president of the United States about one hundred years ago, lived during the Revolutionary War. Asked regarding the capitol of this country, he replied, "The capitol of Chicago is the White House."

On school subjects he was exceedingly deficient in arithmetic, although in this he had been given much training. He added four-place numbers correctly, but very slowly. He failed entirely on an example in long division. He had been studying fractions for some time at school and was having drill in them at the time we saw him, yet he failed on the simplest examples of this type. Nor did he succeed better when reasoning problems were assigned him; thus, he could not tell how much three and one half pounds would cost if two and one half pounds cost forty-five cents. This was true in spite of the fact that the school which he was then attending stressed number work particularly.

His disability in the perception of relationships, in apperception, and reasoning would hardly seem to account for his failure in arithmetic on the rote side, but back of this might have existed an unusual difficulty in acquiring the concept of number, due to his general defect for appreciating relationships. Certain it is that in spite of very good instruction of the usual kind, he has learned comparatively little in this field. What he might have gained, had there been a recognition of his peculiar mental make-up, is a matter of conjecture. One wonders what the results might have been had a special effort been made to have him acquire the concept of number by concrete experience, emphasizing the idea of relationship. Had the underlying principles been grasped, perhaps his good memory powers would then have been of great assistance in this realm as elsewhere.

In their bearing on behavior, Julian's disabilities were exceedingly important. This boy's family had decided that he should become an accountant. They were keeping him in an expensive school with this in view, yet it was just this type of work which was most difficult for him; indeed, it was practically impossible for him to do it well. On his part there was intense dislike of school, which, no doubt, was a factor in the truancy and incorrigibility for which he was noted. Furthermore, this lack of understanding on the part of his family led to irritation at home.

It may be difficult to determine what type of employment this boy is best fitted for; however that may be, we can readily reach the negative conclusion that for some types of work he is undoubtedly not suited. Of course, he was but fourteen when we saw him and was in need of further education, but here, too, the problem arises as to the methods and subjects by which he would profit most. No doubt, it would require much ingenuity to plan in detail a course of study for this boy, but, on the other hand, it would be quite worth while, both for him and for any educator who wished to learn more concerning some intricate, but very practical problems of pedagogy.

Other Disabilities: The above presentation does not include all possible mental disabilities, partly because in the present state of limited knowledge this can not be done.   Among school subjects has been omitted the group of informational studies, such as history and geography, because it is evident that the mental traits involved in learning these subjects are those that have already been considered.

Some mental processes have already been discussed in connection with the more complex activities in which they are elements.   Thus, in presenting defects in number work, as well as defects in reading, I have noted poor powers of auditory perceptions, defective auditory memory, especially for numbers, defective visual memory, extreme inability to form arbitrary associations, and defects in powers of analysis and synthesis.   It would be just as logical, though probably not as helpful, to have discussed these processes just here, but certainly there is no need to retrace the same ground.   Certain mental functions not yet enumerated must be mentioned, however.

First, in regard to *attention*.   Defects in this aspect of mental life will not be illustrated; attention is a function of general applicability and a factor in all performance. As already indicated earlier, in the chapter on Differential Diagnosis, poor powers of concentration and application frequently are concomitants of physical and nervous disorders. Then, too, attention varies so largely with the interest that is felt in various subjects that it is difficult to interpret lack of it seen in the laboratory as a real defect.

Distractibility may be studied by tests designed for the purpose, or judgment may be based upon general observations. In either case it can only be stated that inattention was noted at such and such times and for such and such work. Teachers often render the verdict that a child is progressing unsatisfactorily, not because of general dullness, but because of inability to "pay attention." There are two cautions necessary in such interpretations; on the one hand, the inattention may not be as evident on the playground or elsewhere as in the schoolroom, that is, the difficulty may not be with attention, but with interest. In the second place, sometimes the verdict is altogether false, and the child is inattentive because he is an out-and-out mental defective. We have known more than one instance of such erroneous judgment. Here the lack of attention is only the natural consequence of inability to participate in the schoolroom activities, and is not in any sense evidence of a specialized defect. Hence the greatest care is necessary in reaching a diagnosis regarding defect in powers of attention and persistence.[1]

Nor have individual differences which may exist in *artistic endeavors* been touched upon. From everyday experience one can hardly doubt that there are extreme variations in these fields; whether we are dealing with

[1] Studies dealing with the problem of attention are too numerous to mention in detail. However, the reader might here be referred to a discussion of the entire question by Alfred Mann. ("Zur Psychologie und Psychographie der Aufmerksamkeit." *Zeitschrift für Angewandte Psychologie*, Vol. 8, 1914.) This author presents a detailed analysis of the factors that enter into attention and offers an elaborate psychogram for use in the study of any individual's powers of attention. While he refers to adults, the plan is possible for the study of attention in children of school age.

drawing, painting, dancing, singing, or instrumental music, the range extends from the talented to those exceedingly incapable. While unusual gifts in any of the arts is a matter of great practical significance, defects lead to maladjustments that are not often brought to the clinical psychologist for aid.[1]

Defects in *imagination* and *inventive ability* also are exceedingly complex, and while defects in these powers no doubt lead to important consequences, little is known of the practical implications other than common-sense conclusions. There are few tests with established norms, and experience has not enabled us to make any definite generalizations. These powers are so interwoven with mental representation, foresight, and other processes already mentioned, that they are difficult to differentiate.

While individual differences in *learning ability* are found, some people learning very much more readily than others, the term "learning ability" is too inclusive to allow any general distinctions to be helpful. Extreme defect in learning ability, — or rather defect beyond a certain degree, — is an indication of general defect or feeble-mindedness. Consideration of defects in learning ability for special types of material leads to the very problems that have been discussed throughout this book. The author's general point of view may best be stated by saying that defect in learning ability rests upon inadequate functioning of specific mental processes, and that to discover which process or processes are at fault is the crux of the problem of specialized defect.

[1] While it is hardly in place to cite the literature concerning the arts, it may be mentioned that quite a good deal of experimentation has been carried on in the field of music. There are the studies of Seashore ("The Measurement of a Singer", *Science*, February, 1912) and of Hans Rupp (" Über die Prüfung Musikalischer Fähigkeiten." *Zeitschrift für angewandte Psychologie*, Vol. 9, 1915), who has discussed in detail, methods for testing recognition of pitch, intervals, melody, harmony, time, rhythm, etc.

CHAPTER VIII

DEFECTS IN MENTAL CONTROL

THE psychological elements in the background of voluntary reactions can be quite clearly analyzed.   In general, control of actions is dependent upon control of the mental states leading to actions.   Both emotions and ideas have a very vital relationship to behavior.   Almost all emotions tend to arouse action, while the chief restraining forces lie in the realm of ideas.   Without entering into any discussion of vexed points concerning "the will", it may fairly be said that defective powers of control of actions may be due, on the one hand, to inability to repress the feelings, that is, to lack of emotional control; and, on the other, to failure to arouse inhibiting ideas. From this it may be seen that defective power of control involves both emotional and ideational or volitional aspects of mental life.

The practical issues with which we are here concerned are recognition of the existence of this type of defect and of the need that arises for adjustment of social conditions to meet the responses that such defect calls forth. For, though the general topic of inhibition finds a place in most textbooks on psychology, a rather minor place it must be acknowledged, and though some practical workers have recognized the lack of normal powers of inhibition as a situation with which to reckon, yet the fact that defect in control may be an innate characteris-

166

tic has received almost no recognition by psychologists, nor is it appreciated by many who deal intimately with human beings.

A moment's reflection should convince any one that special defect in control of actions is a phenomenon no more peculiar than is disability of any other type. The power to awaken inhibiting ideas and to keep such thoughts in the foreground of consciousness so that they may become effective, is a power as truly characteristic of mental life as is the capacity for recalling past experience or for performing any other mental function. Then, too, there are, no doubt, inborn differences in the intensity of the emotions as well as in the capacity for resisting emotions, impulses, and desires. Situations apparently the same are in reality quite unlike for different people, arousing feelings so varied and of such different degrees of intensity that the reactions arising therefrom represent necessity for widely varying degrees of control.

Davenport has called individuals showing such defect in powers of control "the feebly inhibited", under which caption he has included three groups; those who display violent temper,[1] those of a hyper- or of a hypo-kinetic temperament, and those who have a tendency towards nomadism.[2] His interest lies chiefly in determining the heritability of such characteristics and the modes of their inheritance. The general explanation of all these so-called types of uncontrolled behavior, according to this author, is "possibly a paralysis of the inhibitory mechanism." These findings cannot here be reviewed critically; that

[1] Davenport, C. B., "The Feebly Inhibited: Violent Temper and Its Inheritance." *Journal of Nervous and Mental Diseases*, September, 1915.

[2] Davenport, C. B., "The Feebly Inhibited: Nomadism or the Wandering Impulse with Special Reference to Heredity." "Carnegie Institute Publication", 536.

would carry us too far afield; but his studies of the subject have strengthened Healy's contention that there are individuals who show innate defects in mental control.

What the inhibitory mechanism, the neural basis of inhibition, may be is discussed in all textbooks dealing with physiological psychology. The general opinion is that nervous impulses are converted into inhibition as truly as into other types of action, for action is restraint as well as movement. "In the mental world, we may suppose that the action of the nervous system may be to check as well as to arouse a sensation or idea. . . . We are men and not brutes because the neurons concerned with the ideational and moral life keep in subjection and counteract the direct impulses to action of the neurones concerned with greed, lust, cruelty, and hatred. We reason and do not simply day-dream, because we can check foolish, irrelevant fancies — can inhibit all ideas that do not lead on to the desired goal." [1] In thinking, at least in purposive thinking, we inhibit and eliminate unfit thoughts; we select and reject in accord with a purpose.

Whether or not it is some flaw in the neural mechanism that accounts for defects in mental control and whatever theories of inheritance of feeble inhibition may prove true, the fact remains that the problems which arise in the case of individuals defective in control are extremely practical. Those who have dealt extensively with delinquents are familiar with the characteristics of this type of individual, their inability to resist temptations, their extreme bad temper, angry threats, and violent reactions.[2]

Following are some examples illustrating this kind of defect:

[1] Thorndike, E. L., "The Elements of Psychology." 1905.
[2] For further discussion, see Healy, "The Individual Delinquent."

Case 32. Social reactions and mental tests both clearly reveal defective powers of control in the case of this girl, otherwise quite normal mentally and physically.

Alice J., 13½ years old, was brought to us by her mother, who stated that she was having a great deal of difficulty in controlling the girl. The mother herself proved to be a very intelligent woman of good judgment and much force of character. She gave a fairly good account of heredity and developmental history, as well as of the troubles which she had experienced with her daughter.

The problem which Alice presented was entirely one of behavior. She had a good record for scholarship, but her deportment had been so objectionable that she had been expelled from school three times. She was said to be quarrelsome with the children and extremely restless in class. In each of the schools she attended — she had been changed frequently — she had been a source of much trouble because of her peculiarly mischievous actions. All together she proved so annoying that the public schools refused to accept her again, and she was even refused the use of one of the city playgrounds. Her mother complained that Alice's erraticism was extreme. She would leave home and ask any stranger that she met for carfare or ask to be taken to a theatre. On one occasion she had visited a friend and while left alone in the room had opened a desk and read the papers which it contained. The family complained that the evenings at home were almost intolerable because of this girl's restlessness and because they never could count upon what she was going to do next. She had almost a mania for dressing herself up and acting a part. In the mother's own words, "Alice dresses up so frequently and changes about so much that it has gotten on the nerves of the whole family." She never remained interested in any one thing for long; if she began to embroider she would soon stop to begin something else in which she would be interested for equally as short a time.

Alice was said to be unlike any member of the family. The heredity, so far as we could learn, was negative. There was said to be no mental trouble of any kind. Special effort was made in this instance to discover any facts regarding the family history which might have a bearing upon the situation. Both parents had always been healthy, except that the mother was greatly worried during this pregnancy because of financial reverses that her husband suffered. For more than a month she was in bed then because of some sort of exhaustion, but we were unable to obtain any accurate diagnosis of what this trouble was. The two older sisters, already married when we saw Alice, were said to be bright and normal in every way, and a younger brother of nine had the reputation of being one of the brightest boys in the school he attended. There had been no difficulties of conduct with them.

The later developmental history regarding Alice was negative. She was said never to have been severely ill. When an infant she had fallen and struck her head, but was said not to have been unconscious. There was, however, history of very frequent enuresis continued until she was eleven or twelve years old. Our examination revealed little of significance. There were no signs of nervous disturbance. The girl was normally developed and well nourished. There were no sensory defects of any kind. The mother insisted that the lack of self-control was already noticeable when Alice was only three years of age.

The psychological examination showed numerous peculiarities, both on test results and on incidental reactions. We soon were convinced that Alice had quite good innate ability. The simpler tests which could be done rapidly were done correctly. Construction tests were solved by trial and error method. She showed little deliberation before beginning a test, starting pell-mell, trying almost anything, but showing a capacity to profit by her own errors. The record on the apperception tests was normal, and she did the learning tests readily. The poorest results were obtained on the tapping test, where very defective psychomotor control was shown. Either she worked very slowly, or when an effort was made to increase speed many errors were made. On memory tests there was quite a difference between those for rote memory and logical passages. The former were done quite well, the latter very poorly. It was evident that this was due to poor powers of attention and lack of steadiness of purpose. Many of the items were omitted, many changes were made, and there was no adherence to logical sequence. In school work she was fairly well advanced, showing ability to do well the work of the seventh grade.

More striking than test results was her behavior on the several occasions when we ourselves had an opportunity to observe her. In the laboratory Alice was never quiet long. She handled constantly any of the material within reach, and was playing with one thing or another incessantly. She showed extreme curiosity, but even this wavered; before she had examined any one object thoroughly she had already picked up something else. This poor control in attention was evident in test work too; in the beginning she would look at the examiner, apparently paying very close attention, but sometimes, when half through a task, her mind seemed to wander and she centered her attention on something else. On the emotional side she was equally uncontrolled. Once during the testing she grasped the examiner quite convulsively and began to sob, explaining this by the fact that a question asked her had recalled some unpleasant experience. A moment later she was laughing in regard to some other idea which had been suggested to her.

Dismissed from the room for a few moments while her mother was being consulted, she came back crying because she had seen a little girl who had no mother. She wanted immediately to take this girl home. Soon, however, she was laughing, quite forgetful of her new friend's bad fortune. Later we were informed that while she was out of the room she had investigated all the cabinets in the outer office, had walked down the hall of the building in which the laboratory is situated, talking to every one she met. We ourselves soon witnessed her inordinate curiosity and her uncontrolled manner of investigating everything in her vicinity; she peered into the desk and other places, sitting still for only a minute or two at a time. In her conversation she was rather flighty, giving statements that were not to be relied upon. She told us that her parents were Protestant and immediately after said they were not.

We were unable to find any hidden conflict or worry. In spite of her forward manner and extreme friendliness in approaching strangers she had not met with any bad experiences, and whatever she had heard from bad companions left her mind as fast as it entered, according to the mother, with whom Alice seemed to have a very nice and confidential relationship.

We have here, then, a girl normal as regards intelligence, but decidedly defective in self-control. In every way she shows her lack in normal powers of inhibition. Her mental processes seem totally uncontrolled, her word is unreliable, she will say anything that comes into her mind. As for her emotions, they are volatile, changing from moment to moment, and thoroughly unstable. Her behavior at school and at home clearly indicates the fact that the girl acts upon any impulse that presents itself. She does not inhibit these even when they lead to conduct which she knows will injure her. In spite of coming from a cultured home, the girl was poorly informed and showed a paucity of mental interests, the lack quite possibly being the result of her flighty mental processes. Taking into account the history given by the mother and the officer who knew the case well, the observations of her general behavior, her conversation, and her work on psychological tests, one could only conclude that this was a case of defect in mental control, and that there was no evident physical basis for it.

The seriousness of this defect and the social significance of it are very apparent. Such a girl might easily get into any kind of trouble on the city streets. Her behavior is so unaccountable, she is so much the victim of her own impulses, that it would be impossible to predict what might or might not occur. Only one of two things offer themselves in such a case: The girl could be placed in a special institution for nervous children where her environment would be controlled and where perhaps she could be given good discipline, or the parents would have to endeavor to exert this discipline themselves, aiding her in every way to acquire self-control. In this instance the mother was a very capable woman and a good disciplinarian. It was advised that the family move out to the suburbs, where it would be quieter and safer for the girl, and that the mother keep close watch over her. It seemed quite possible that with advancing age and 'her own better understanding of the problem, the girl might develop stronger powers of inhibition.

Since we first studied this case we have received frequent reports. The erratic type of behavior has not altogether ceased, but gradually there has been improvement, and now, after a lapse of two years, Alice has entered high school and has a fair record there. She is said to be still quite uncontrolled, and her word is not regarded as altogether reliable, but her peculiar reactions are less extreme, and she is becoming more conscious of their import and making an effort to control herself better.

Case 33. Here defect in control of actions rests probably on an unstable nervous organization due to many early illnesses. In this case lack of mental control is plainly shown on tests.

Morgan G., 14 years old, had been brought to us with a query as to what could be done for the boy. The officer who was interested in the case felt that he would not be accepted again in school, since his record there had been so unsatisfactory. He was said by his teachers to be extremely troublesome. He was restless, into petty mischief, and so flighty and erratic in his general behavior that some teachers had considered him feebleminded. He had only reached the third grade. It was reported that he did no work in school unless constantly watched. For a short period after leaving school he had tried to get employment, but employers would not keep him. They said that the boy was erratic and exceedingly talkative, and too uncontrolled in his general behavior. While Morgan had never been an extreme delinquent, yet he had proven troublesome everywhere. The mother made the same type of complaint regarding him, but she herself was compelled to work away from home all day and probably had never exercised very good oversight or discipline.

In regard to heredity, very little was known about the boy's father or the father's family. The father had died before this child was born, and the mother had never even met her husband's relatives. As for her family, there was no history of any mental trouble, except that, of fourteen siblings, one developed epilepsy and later insanity.

The mother had not been well during the pregnancy, and when the child was born instruments were used, and the head was much marked. The mother maintained that a scar was visible until he was about ten years old, but no indications of any head injury were apparent at the time of our physical examination. As a baby he was sickly, had marasmus, and weighed only seven pounds when thirteen months old. He had frequent convulsions from the first to the tenth month but none later. He suffered from many illnesses, pneumonia three times, measles, diphtheria, and whooping cough. He first walked and talked when between two and three years old.

When we saw the boy we found him to have several poor physical conditions, though his general development was good, and he was well nourished. His vision was somewhat defective, tonsils were moderately enlarged, there was a severe valvular lesion with slight enlargement of the heart. There were no nervous disorders of any kind. He had bright eyes and quite normal expression.

Mental examination was interesting and significant. In the laboratory Morgan's general characteristics, as given by his teacher, his mother, and the probation officer, were quite apparent. He seemed restless, ever on the alert, anxious to begin a test before complete directions had been given, persistent in his efforts for a short time, and then unable to give very close attention. Where tests particularly required good mental control he had much difficulty, and, once confused regarding the solution of a problem, he became hopelessly lost. There was a very marked difference in the performance of tests of different types. He did all the Binet tests through twelve years satisfactorily and without any trouble, showing on these and other tests that he was normal in his general ability. The more difficult construction test was done without any trouble, whereas in doing the simpler one he became much confused and failed entirely to solve it. When, however, it was given him again about an hour later, he solved it immediately by a very rational process. We found nothing peculiar in his memory processes nor in his general powers of apperception. On the other hand, all tests for mental control were performed poorly. He showed extreme difficulty in the control of his verbal associations; in giving the opposites to simple words the time varied considerably from word to word. Again, on the continuous subtraction test, he showed even more strikingly this characteristic lack of mental control. He was utterly unable to subtract seven continuously from one hundred, although able to perform much more difficult work than this in written arithmetic of the ordinary type. When endeavoring to subtract by fours from forty-one he began very well, but' after a few seconds he found it so difficult to keep his mind upon the problem that he made most absurd failures and eventually had to subtract by ones, counting backwards until he had subtracted four numbers. Doing this, he made no error in subtraction until he reached the number twenty-five, after which he said "four from twenty-five is twenty, four from twenty is twenty-eight", and no one other combination after this was correct. He realized that he was incorrect, but in spite of an effort to do better he steadily grew worse. Nor did the boy show good psychomotor control. In the tapping test he was both slow and inaccurate.

As for his school work, we found that he was able to do long division, that he wrote simple sentences quite well, and could read about a third-grade passage with good expression, although in a rather jerky manner. It was

quite evident that he was able to master the ordinary
school subjects, and that the low grade he had reached
must therefore have been due to the disciplinary features
of the case. We have no doubt that his defect in control of his mental processes interfered very seriously with
his school life and was also the explanation of his erratic,
uncontrolled behavior. The boy was not at all vicious.
He was a friendly lad, who apparently wished to do his
best and to get on with people, but the peculiarities of
his mental processes were such that it was difficult for
him to behave like the average child.

It can well be imagined that such a boy would present
a difficult problem in the ordinary classroom. In group
work with others he would no doubt be the source of a
good deal of commotion and be regarded by his teachers
as a nuisance. His very friendliness, coupled with his
lack of self-control, made him, no doubt, the great talker
that he was reputed to be. These characteristics would
be a great handicap in ordinary kinds of employment.
In most of the positions available in the city, particularly
such as an uneducated boy could fill, his innate traits
would be most undesirable.

We later had a striking example of this boy's typical
reactions. Upon our recommendation that his eyes and
throat be examined by specialists he was taken to a
hospital, where his tonsils were removed. Then he was
returned to the institution in which we had studied the
case. The nurse in charge found him a most trying
patient during his convalescence. He was ever into some
mischief, was most difficult to keep occupied and quiet,
and one day having lost her patience, the nurse had re-
marked — not, of course, seriously — "You are just too
bad to live, you are such a lot of trouble." The idea of
dying having been suggested to the boy, he thereupon
really endeavored to commit suicide by strangling him-

self. From a later conversation with him we learned that the boy had not been at all despondent, nor desirous of ending his life; the idea of suicide having come to him, he did not control or inhibit the thought, but acted speedily upon it.

It is difficult to offer a prognosis in the case of this lad. Of course, he should have all the help possible in correction of his physical disabilities, and we advised that after this was done he be placed at a farm school, where he would have some academic training, but where a good part of his day would be spent in open-air activities. The greatest hope lies in bettering his physical conditions and in developing his apperceptions of his own difficulties, so that he can, and perhaps will, make a greater effort to control himself.

Case 34. We have here an illustration of defective powers of inhibition correlated with poor mental and psychomotor control as indicated by results on tests. In this case the physical conditions were splendid.

Henry B., 17 years old, had been in the United States six or seven years, having come from a country district in Austria. He had learned English quite well, had progressed satisfactorily at school, and when we knew him was in court for the first time. He had been brought to us by his parents, who maintained that they could not tolerate him at home because of his violent temper. He behaved so badly that there had been several complaints of disturbance made by the neighbors. His general incorrigibility had increased until recently he had thrown his father to the floor and was in the act of beating him when the police were called.

We learned that the boy had been a source of disturbance in the home for a long time, but he had not been guilty of any other type of misconduct than that shown there. All complaints had been of the same character, namely, about his exceeding violence, his high temper, and his inability to get along with people. Later we came to know about this boy's behavior in a very good secondary school to which he had been sent. He got in various petty troubles with classmates, and finally was asked to leave because of his fighting and quarrelsomeness.

We found this boy to be immensely big and broad shouldered, overdeveloped physically and premature in sex development. Except for slight tremor of outstretched hands, the physical findings were negative.

The main characteristic shown on psychological tests was his exceeding lack of mental control. Considering the fact that he had not attended school in his native land, he had done well here in book work. He had completed the sixth grade and then had gone to a private school, where his record for scholarship was fair enough. Noting in detail his work on psychological tests, we found that he did construction tests very well. The so-called cross line tests for mental analysis were done correctly; the pictorial apperception test was also well done, no illogical errors being made. He graded as normal on Binet tests. His memory powers were good and tests for reasoning were likewise satisfactorily performed. He followed simple directions well, but made a rather poor record on the difficult directions test, where perhaps the "catches" were not recognized because the wording of them would be quite involved for one whose knowledge of English was not particularly good.

In contradistinction to the number of things on which he did well, the results on tests for mental control were very poor indeed. The record on the tapping test was poor both for speed and accuracy; control of verbal associations was notably lacking; the reactions on the opposites test were irregular, there were quite a few errors made and the time varied greatly from word to word. In the continuous subtraction test numerous peculiarities were noted. The more difficult portion, at least where the numbers involved are larger, was correctly done, but as he went on, the boy became confused and himself said, "I get mixed up." In each of three efforts many errors were made.

In his general reactions while working with tests, we noted the same lack of control. He was most eager to make a good record. He was very talkative while he was working, but his remarks were not always relevant. He would say one thing when he meant another, correct himself, and at times become almost incoherent. Later, in telling the story of the troubles which led to his arrest, he became quite excited and less coherent than ever.

Neither the hereditary nor the developmental history is well known in regard to Henry, the parents in their broken English gave a rather meager account, but the type of difficulties in which he has been involved is interesting in the light of the findings on tests alone. It can readily be seen from even our brief statement that, although this boy is fairly well endowed in intelligence and rather unusually well endowed physically, he cannot be regarded as altogether normal in regard to his mental life. Here the defect is clearly one of control. It seems clear that there is distinct relationship between this lack of mental control and his social behavior.

Case 35. The following is an instance of defective powers of inhibition where extreme lack of control of the emotions is shown, but no abnormal reactions were found on tests for mental control.

Celia K., 17 years old when first seen, had been brought into court for sex delinquency. She was held awaiting trial, but a short time before it was perceived by all who came in contact with her that she was an extremely

troublesome girl, difficult to manage. From the super-
intendent, school teacher, and various attendants came
similar bad reports. Celia frequently had periods of
violent temper lasting two or three hours, during which
she appeared capable of almost any misconduct. On
one occasion she broke the panel of a door to pieces;
in the schoolroom she threw articles of furniture about,
quarreled with the girls, became easily angered, and
when angry expressed herself in the coarsest of language.
Following a period of this kind she was generally found
quivering and white. She herself said that after she had
been excited and given way to her temper she felt faint
and weak, that during her excitement she actually did
not know where she was part of the time.

Celia showed herself on all occasions to be extremely
self-willed. She freely acknowledged her own wilfulness,
and when it was explained to her that her conduct would
result in injury to her own case, she merely replied she
did not care what happened to her and that she would
do as she pleased. In the court room she behaved very
badly, creating a disturbance by her lack of self-control.

Later she was sent to a correctional institution for
girls. There she soon earned a reputation in consonance
with her earlier behavior and was regarded as being
insane. Because of this she was returned for further
study. When discussing the situation with us, she behaved in a most foolish manner, refusing to view the
matter as anything serious; she laughed and grinned
much, spoke flippantly and exceedingly volubly. Her
explanation was that when she liked people and they
treated her well she got on without trouble, but if any
one treated her unjustly or harshly she lost all control of
herself, and said and did things for which she felt herself
to be hardly accountable. Our own experience showed
that even her likes were expressed in uncontrolled fashion;

if she took a fancy to a person she would express it in a very demonstrative manner.

Later, after having been released from the institution, Celia returned home, but before long proved herself uncontrollable, became once more involved in sex delinquencies, and was returned to the court. Thereupon she was again sent to an institution. For a time things went very well, then something occurred which she felt was unjust and she fought so strenuously against discipline that was meted out to her and behaved so tempestuously that once more she was placed under our observation for mental diagnosis. At this time the girl was in a very serious mood; she told us that on her second commitment she had resolved to make great efforts to behave herself and earn a good record, but in spite of earnest endeavor, she failed under unusual stress.

From her mother we learned that Celia had frequently been untruthful and unreliable. She claimed once that she was working when this was not true and had invented a story altogether fictitious when first arrested. Previously she had run away from home without any particular provocation. She had always been regarded as exceedingly lazy. After leaving school she did not wish to work, and earlier, while still attending school, she had made little effort to learn. We were never able to obtain a school record and do not know whether Celia was a disciplinary problem there or not. We know that she was not interested in school work, that she took little advantage of such educational opportunities as were offered her, but this, too, may have been due to her general lack of self-control.

The facts of heredity and family history were not altogether satisfactorily obtained, for the mother was only fairly intelligent and though anxious to coöperate she knew little concerning her husband's family. Both parents were foreign born and poorly educated. Celia's father had not worked for eleven years. He claimed to be ill, but in reality he was probably merely lazy. He had been alcoholic previously. The mother, who had worked for a number of years in order to support the family, was apparently a good woman. We could learn of no mental trouble in either family. Celia had walked and talked early, had been a healthy child, had suffered no illnesses except measles when ten years old. The physical examination showed the girl to be exceedingly big and strong, a vivacious, active type. Vision was somewhat defective, teeth very badly in need of attention, and there was a partial nasal occlusion. The girl complained of headaches, but we could get no history of any form of attacks. She was not over-developed in physical sex characteristics.

As for psychological examination, the results were interesting and very definite. As we expected from what had been told us, we found that Celia could do little in the way of school work. Although born in America, she had never attended English-speaking schools, and English was not spoken in the home; aside from these disadvantages, there was no doubt that she had not endeavored to learn and might have gained much more from routine school work had she made an effort to do so. She understood the fundamental processes of arithmetic, but was inaccurate in the use of them. She could write only a few simple words and her reading of English was exceedingly poor. She failed on the longer words of even a first-grade passage; this may mean little, for she had received little training in English.

On the other hand, she graded as normal by Binet tests. She did performance tests quite well and showed normal powers of apperception. Even on tests for mental control the results were good, but it must be remembered that she realized the import of the examination, understanding full well that our verdict regarding her mentality would be of vital importance in the disposition of her case. In consequence, no doubt, she made a very decided effort. Besides this, she was friendly in her attitude towards us, believing that we were desirous of helping her. Occasionally, with all her effort to control her mental processes, she would laugh, or rather simper, foolishly during the examination. Her powers of psychomotor control were not good.

Here, again, although we have no tests for quantitative measurement, we know that there was poor emotional control. Her behavior at home, during detention, and even while under special observation, indicated this. She herself realized her lack of self-control and was able to state very clearly that this was the root of all her trouble.

When last seen, after her serious difficulty with the institutional authorities, Celia's attitude had changed greatly. She appreciated the fact that her outbreaks of temper led many to consider her aberrational, and that some observers had suggested her transfer to a State institution for the insane. In consequence she seemed very genuine in her intentions to improve her conduct. She herself stated that it would be a hard struggle to master her temper and impulses, but she hoped that perhaps she might succeed in achieving better control. Of course, we felt this to be barely possible and yet feared that, considering the innate defect, there would be failure in spite of good resolutions.

In such a case as this one can hardly hope for a tremendous change in reactions, and a favorable prognosis is less likely in the light of too few mental interests. Of course, Celia is not altogether incapable and even at her age new interests might be awakened. Then, her physical defects should be attended to, for they may be the cause of some irritation, and, above all, she needs outlets for her extreme emotions. She is so big and strong that she really requires hard manual work on which to expend her energies, and probably farm life away from city temptations and offering an opportunity for abundant outdoor occupations would give her the best chance of mastering herself.

On the basis of long observation and repeated testing, we could never reach the conclusion, suggested by others, that Celia was either feeble-minded or insane. Her conversation was altogether too coherent and her self-orientation and apperception of her own innate defects too keen to warrant one in believing that there was any aberration. Rather, her conduct had to be explained on the basis of innately poor emotional control.

Case 36. This case is offered because the behavior of the girl indicates so clearly the innately defective powers of control.

Julia D. is a girl whom we have seen repeatedly over a period of three years. When we first knew her at about 15 years of age, she was already giving much trouble and she has continued to be incorrigible up to the present time. She was first brought to the court by her mother, who declared the girl could not be controlled at home. On several occasions she had run away; she had been exceedingly disobedient and quarrelsome. Not until much later did the girl become a sex delinquent, but, once having begun this delinquency, she became extreme in it. She has been arrested repeatedly. During the three years we have known her she has been placed on probation several times under different officers, and each one of them has felt herself unequal to cope with the girl. So undisciplined and uncontrolled is Julia that it has been suggested more than once that she must be insane, but this, as we shall see later, was shown not to be true.

Held in detention pending her appearance at court her record was exceedingly bad. She had violent spells of temper. On one occasion, without any known provocation, while at the supper table, she threw a cup at another girl. At times she refused to eat with the others and then later demanded food because she was hungry. In the schoolroom she was a source of great annoyance and disturbance. If things did not suit her, she would throw chairs and other things, and once she lifted a chair to strike another girl. There was hardly a person in the girl's department with whom she did not fight. She was notorious for her use of bad language.

In the court, where it surely was to her advantage to control herself and behave properly, she showed the same kind of unfortunate reactions. When a suggestion was made which did not meet with her approval, she shrieked, threw herself on the floor, and created a terrible scene.

At the institution for girls to which she was sent she exhibited exactly the same traits. She behaved so badly that it was felt impossible to keep her there, — a result which she may have desired. However, when placed on probation with the understanding that if she behaved herself properly she would not only be allowed to remain at liberty but would be helped to obtain a position, she continued her violently delinquent behavior, and it was necessary to bring her back into court. At this time it was noted that the girl seemed most sincere in her promise to try to do better than previously.

When first examined, Julia was a small and rather poorly developed girl; she appeared, however, quite healthy. There were no sensory defects of any kind, and nothing significant was noted on the physical side other than her excessive frowning and very surly expression.

We were unable to get an altogether satisfactory

account of the heredity. We knew the father to be an
exceedingly brutal man, who beat his children, and who
seemed to feel that their greatest obligation to him was
in the matter of their supporting him. The mother evidently was under his influence, and the home conditions
were very bad. There was a large family. Eventually
the mother left the father and returned to Europe, where
her parents still resided. Among the siblings we noted
that there was no mental trouble. Two older sisters
had been in court, but the delinquencies of neither one
had been at all extreme, and bad home conditions sufficiently explained the misconduct. One of these girls
has turned out very well indeed; the other has become a
great sex delinquent. We have never been able to learn
that either was given to violent outbreaks of temper or
to any other form of violent or uncontrolled behavior.

Julia was said never to have been very sick and to have
developed normally. She had, of course, been thrown in
contact with the delinquent older sisters and later with
other bad companions, but it could hardly be alleged that
these were very great influences, for she herself was much
more a leader than a follower. Her outbreaks of violence were not based upon any conflicts or hidden emotional disturbance, so far as we were able to learn.

As previously stated, some have considered this girl
insane, particularly those who have seen her in one of
her fits of temper. For this reason a very thorough psychological examination was originally made, and Julia
was examined again after an interval of two years. We
have always found the girl well oriented; she quite
understood the home situation and her relation to it;
she talked coherently and cogently; she knew well that
she had an ungovernable temper and acknowledged that
she could not control it. There was nothing indicative
of delusions or, indeed, of any form of aberration.

The interesting feature shown on psychological examination was that this girl was able to perform tests for mental control very well indeed. She proved herself to have good innate ability. Performance tests were done rapidly, the records made being better than the average. She had no difficulty in tests for mental analysis; the pictorial apperception test was done without a single error; control of verbal associations was normal; continuous subtraction test was done without an error and fairly rapidly. As for school work, Julia had completed the seventh grade in the public school at thirteen years. Indeed, judged merely by the results on tests nothing of significance would have been noted.

The only conclusion that one can reach in regard to such a problem is that there exists an innate defect in control, that powers of inhibition are not normal. There was no indication of any physical cause for this lack, nor was any explanation gained through study of various mental activities. The emotional make-up cannot be adequately studied by any means now at our disposal; we can only draw inferences in regard to emotions from general behavior. Certainly, in this case the emotions do not seem normal, but the girl never showed any extreme emotional reactions other than her bad temper. Often as we have seen her, we have never known her to cry, to show any violent hatred, or any tendency towards moodiness.

In regard to the influence of adolescence, we recognize the fact that this girl had entered upon that period when she was first seen, but we must also remember that as she grows older her self-control is not becoming any greater; if it were purely an adolescent phenomenon one would expect her to become more stable and better controlled with advancing years. Recent developments in her career give no indication of any betterment of behavior; a short time ago, the girl escaped from a correctional institution, engaged in extreme immorality and stealing, was sent once more to a correctional institution, this time to one for adults. Upon her release, after a short sentence there, she attempted suicide; the exact events leading to this act we do not know.

Now we can only regard the outlook for the future as extremely doubtful. As in the previous case, we had earlier advised the development of better mental interests, and removal to a quieter environment. Unfortunately, this advice could never be followed; even now it offers the best chance that remains for any possible improvement.

Case 37. Here, again, we note great lack of control in the case of a boy well endowed mentally and physically, but who nevertheless is an extreme delinquent, mainly, it would seem, because of his innate defect in emotional control.

Oliver L., at 17 years of age a big, well developed young fellow, was first brought into court a number of years before the case was studied by us. Indeed, from the court records we note that he was already proving troublesome when ten years old, at which time he was sent out to the country. No sooner was he returned to the city than he was again delinquent. In the intervening years his record for behavior was poor and since we have seen him he has been still further delinquent. He is regarded by all who know him as exceedingly unreliable. Not only is he notoriously untruthful, but reports from his various places of employment show him to be unstable in his general behavior. On one occasion, for instance, when he was expected to come to court he did not appear, although from previous experience he knew this would reflect badly upon him. In explanation he weakly told the judge that he intended to report after he had gotten a job, and did not think that there was any harm in waiting a few days.

After graduating from grammar school he worked at a number of occupations. Because he is a strong, nice looking boy of good intelligence, he has had little difficulty in obtaining one position after another. Most of them he has voluntarily relinquished after working only a short time. The family report that he is troublesome in every way at home. He is in general lazy; he remains out late nights in spite of their efforts to keep him occupied and happy at home. At various times he has left home and traveled about the country. On one occasion he went to New York, stayed there two hours, and then, although he had never been there previously, returned home. Speaking of this, he later said he really had no desire to see the city, he did not suppose it any different from other cities, and, besides, he wanted to "move on." It was then that he suddenly made up his mind to journey to Florida. He has also been to the Pacific coast, always making his own way. At times Oliver has given way extensively to bad sex habits, occasionally with other boys, but most often when alone.

Aside from the record of delinquency the most notable feature in regard to this boy's behavior is his remarkable lack of control of his emotions; for example, even in the courtroom, when quite a few persons were present, he broke down in the midst of his story and cried bitterly. This seemed such peculiar behavior for a big, strong fellow of his age, that it was the occasion of our being asked to study the boy.

We found him physically in exceedingly good condition. There were no sensory defects nor any other physical findings of significance. As for mentality, we soon were confident that the boy had very good mental powers. He did a wide range of tests very well indeed. Abstract

material was handled as successfully as concrete. Tests
for mental control were performed normally; even the
code test was easy for him. But in the laboratory, as
elsewhere, we were impressed with the lack of control
of his emotions. No sooner was any topic concerning
himself touched upon than the boy drew down the cor-
ners of his mouth and began to cry. Indeed, he wept so
bitterly that it was difficult for him to continue work for
quite a long time. The same reaction was noted over and
over on various occasions and in the presence of different persons.

The family history was given us by an older brother,
a very successful business man, quite well educated, and
fine in his attitude toward the delinquent boy. From
him we learned that the heredity was altogether negative. The father, dead a number of years, had been a
very good man, not alcoholic, and a very hard worker;
he was a member of a family in which there was no mental
trouble. The mother we found to be a very good woman;
she had never heard of epilepsy or insanity in any member of her family. Of the three siblings, Oliver was the
only one who had ever caused any trouble. This older
brother and an older sister had graduated from school
with good records, both were married, and had never
been in trouble of any kind. Oliver had always been
healthy, in fact, unusually so. He had gone to school
at the usual age, had been considered a bright boy, but
early was in trouble and was once expelled. He was said
to have associated with bad companions to quite a great
extent, but no one of them had a record equal to his own.
An interesting feature which came to light was the fact
that the boy very frequently was penitent and many
times had sincerely promised to do better, but invariably
fell back into his old ways.

We have here, then, an example of a boy strong and well

physically, mentally quite capable, who is lacking, however, in normal control of his emotions, and who shows
his instability and poor powers of inhibition by his social
reactions. There is no adequate explanation of his
delinquencies other than his innate defect. Here the
misconduct began prior to adolescence and has continued
over a long period. One can only hope that with advancing age the boy will be able to exert better control through
a deeper appreciation of the necessity for this. (As a
matter of fact, our later reports show that this boy is
slowly improving.)

Case 38. To illustrate the fact that defects in mental
and emotional control may be so excessive as to verge
upon a psychosis, we cite the following case.

Allen B., nearly 13 years of age, was seen when brought
by his parents, who complained that his behavior at home
was excessively uncontrolled. His older sister reported
that he swore terribly, that recently he had chased his
mother with a knife, shrieking at her and calling her the
worst of names, merely because his bed had been shifted
a little. He had on several occasions attempted to
attack his mother; once he had gathered stones to throw
at her; he had beaten his father; fought with the brothers
and sisters, calling them insulting names in the presence of
visitors; refused to eat what was prepared for the family; on one occasion in a rage he had run away from home
several blocks on the city streets clad only in his under-
garments. Though poor, the family had tried to humor
him and had bought a violin hoping that he would become interested in music, for which he seemed to have
talent. They paid fifty dollars for the instrument, and
Allen in a fit of temper broke it to pieces. The teacher
who had come to the house was driven out by the boy.
A long recital of misconduct was to the effect that the
boy exhibited extreme temper and lack of control. His

people felt that he was dangerous, and something must be done in the home situation.

The family history showed that Allen came from extremely neurotic and psychopathic stock. The mother was very nervous, always excitable, and easily frightened. The father, a very hard-working man, was asthmatic and otherwise sickly; he was extremely irritable, complaining constantly, and never was known to smile or appear happy. An older sister was excessively nervous; she had fainting attacks and became easily frightened, at which time she would tremble all over; she told us of attacks of dizziness and of early chorea; the greater part of three years during adolescence she had spent in a hospital. Another sister, bright in school, likewise showed nervous signs which had been diagnosed as chorea.

We could learn nothing significant regarding the developmental history of Allen. He had a good school record, was in the seventh grade. He was said to prepare his lessons regularly, and his conduct was considerably better at school than at home. Physically he was rather small for his age and poorly developed. He complained of headaches and of vertigo when he read too long, but vision was not very defective as judged by a rough examination; however, we felt that he should have his eyes studied by a specialist. He did not drink tea or coffee to excess, did not smoke, and was not known to have any bad habits. In all other respects physical examination was negative. There were no indications of nervous disturbance; reflexes were quite normal, no tremors noted.

As for mentality, it was most difficult to reach any conclusion because of the peculiarities of the lad. His general lack of self-control was most apparent upon testing him. He would, perhaps, begin an interview in a very friendly manner, showing the greatest willingness to coöperate, but might soon change his mood. In the midst of one test he became hysterical, laughing in a most uncontrolled manner over the absurdities test of the Binet series. Whenever he did not see the solution of a problem quickly, he became utterly confused and hopelessly involved. Thus, on one of the construction tests, his record was extremely poor; on each of two trials he failed to solve this. His powers of apperception, as indicated by tests as well as by his behavior, were decidedly poor. He made seven errors out of possible ten, on the pictorial apperception test, although a normal twelve-year-old boy should be able to perform this satisfactorily. His lack of good mental control was further indicated in a reading test, where he read the selection fluently, but in the reproduction incorporated ideas of his own which changed the meaning altogether.

Seen a second day, the boy once more began well, but when he made a poor record on a certain test, his expression changed to one of intense moroseness; he refused to do any further work and began to cry. An effort was made on a third day, at which time it was found that he had extremely poor control of his verbal associations, since he made 7 errors in giving the opposites to 20 different words. About a week later the boy once more came to the laboratory and this time succeeded with several tests on which he had previously failed, but the opposites test for control of associations and the apperception test were as poorly done as formerly.

Our final diagnosis regarding the mentality of this boy was that he was a border-line case of psychosis. That he was innately capable was shown by his good school record and by the ease with which he passed all of the Binet tests for general intelligence, but his lack of mental control was equally as apparent. His reactions on numerous tests showed decidedly aberrational tendencies, and his behavior indicated his defect in powers of inhibition and control. In this instance, of course, the hereditary basis was obvious.

One can scarcely see how such a boy could get on in the family environment. It was recommended that he be placed in a quiet country home where there would be less in the way of irritation and more in the way of good discipline. We bore in mind, of course, that the aberrational tendencies might increase, and the boy might develop an out-and-out psychosis. However, while the family showed such extreme neurotic tendencies and lack of nervous stability, none of them had ever been really insane.

CHAPTER IX

SPECIAL ABILITIES WITH GENERAL MENTAL SUB-NORMALITY

WHEREAS this book has previously dealt with types of special disabilities found in individuals otherwise normal mentally, in this chapter will be considered the opposite type of mental irregularities, namely, special abilities which rise above the level of general mental subnormality. Remembering the definitions and limitations given in the first chapter, we need but reiterate here that we shall confine ourselves to issues which have practical significance in relation to educational and social problems.

One might, of course, discuss special abilities found in the normal, and unusual gifts as seen in the genius or supernormal. But there is a peculiar advantage in studying aptitudes that arise from a level lower than the normal. Because all other powers are defective, the special ability looms large and is therefore more clearly discerned as a separate function. Knowledge derived from study of simpler forms of mental activity is needed to aid in understanding the highly complicated admixture of powers that genius generally represents. Indeed, the type of research presented in this chapter should be greatly extended in the future, that all the unitary functions and powers may be known.

The cases offered in illustration of special abilities do not belong to the group of defectives who can do only the simplest work under direction and who must, therefore, be constantly protected and in many instances permanently segregated. A few are included who grade quite low on the Binet scale and hence would be regarded by some as definitely feeble-minded. However, they give evidence of special abilities of such social significance that there is a strong possibility of successful adjustment to conditions outside an institution. With the emphasis that is now placed on the social definition of the term feeble-minded, many of these individuals could not be committed to a State institution for mental defectives. Their greatest happiness and society's best interests can be most largely conserved by discovering the tasks for which such persons are best fitted and by directing educational and vocational efforts accordingly.

The belief seems quite general that all mental defectives are best fitted for handwork, that their main training should be in the sensory and perceptual fields. A certain amount of the three R's is added to this in the case of those who seem capable of grasping such subjects. What the author would here maintain is that for high grade defectives it is necessary to undertake psychological studies that are intensive, in order to find any special abilities which may exist, since even among defectives capacities are often uneven.

We know from actual experience that not all feeble-minded are adapted to education on the motor side. In illustration, the following instance is cited.

Case 39. A boy of 13 years was graded according to Binet as $7\frac{2}{5}$ years mentally. He was unable to reply to any common-sense questions; memory span for numerals presented either auditorily or visually was distinctly low (four and five numerals respectively). He could not reproduce with any semblance of correctness a passage read to him which contained twelve ideas; his power of association for arbitrary symbols was exceedingly poor;

in the simple substitution test he made five errors, and in a number of other tests, which we need not here enumerate in detail, the results corroborated the Binet findings. There was no doubt that the boy was feeble-minded. On tests for psychomotor control and on construction tests requiring perception of form, or relationships of form, he made extremely poor records. At $11\frac{1}{2}$ years he was unable to copy a diamond shaped figure; he failed on the simple construction test when it was first given him, though he later learned to do this. He failed likewise on the more difficult construction test and on the puzzle box. Given a problem involving concrete material he showed not only the greatest lack of rational procedure in the solution, but even inability to profit by errors when employing a trial and error method. Many impossibilities were tried and repeated; indeed, this boy was poorer in such tests than are many feeble-minded of even lower grade than he.

He had no ability in the handling of numbers; he could only count slowly by ones. However, he showed quite a facility for reading. To our great surprise he was able to render quite fluently a third-grade passage and to reproduce the content fairly well. Considering his limited training in reading, this seemed most remarkable. His special ability was so narrow and unrelated to other mental traits that perhaps little could be made of it in the way of practical application. On the other hand, the chance for training this boy to become an industrial worker with concrete material would seem to be almost nil.

Special ability for some one type of performance is frequently found in members of the subnormal group. It would seem worth while to differentiate the training given to such individuals, at least in specific instances where findings on tests offer justification for it. Those who have particular ability in the field of language could certainly profit by training which would be useless for others. Again, there are some few who, because of special ability for numbers, could perhaps be trained for an occupation where their special gift could be used, rather than have the major portion of their time consumed by training in basketry or other handwork. Sometimes there is a special talent for music, or some other form of art, such as drawing or dancing, or dramatic expression. Or it is an exceptionally good memory, perhaps specialized visual memory or rote memory in general, that stands above the general level of other powers. More often still, there is ability to deal with the concrete, for experience corroborates, on the whole, such studies as Norsworthy's,[1] where it was found that in the sensory fields the normal and the defective are much more nearly equal in ability than in powers of reasoning, judgment, or ability to deal with abstractions. Indeed, some subnormals, and even some feeble-minded, are superior to many a normal person in the doing of handwork. Nor do we mean the very rarely met feeble-minded person with exceptional mechanical and constructive genius.

Occasionally, unusually good motor dexterity may be the exceptional gift, without corresponding skill in manual work. We have long known the case of a young man, now eighteen years old, a mental defective who never did well on tests with concrete material, who has become a very successful boxer. His motor reactions are quick and well controlled, and this, together with his aggressiveness and general forcefulness, makes him something of an expert in his own field.

In apperceptive ability subnormals as well as lower grade defectives vary greatly. We have seen both high-grade morons and border-line individuals who were well

[1] Norsworthy, Naomi. "The Psychology of Mentally Deficient Children." *Archives of Psychology,* 1, 1906.

aware of their own limitations, and then we have seen others who did not appreciate their lack of mental endowment to any adequate degree. Probably the social success of subnormals and high-grade feeble-minded is in direct proportion to the degree of apperceptive ability which they possess; or, at least, this added to other special abilities.

For the final determination of many moot points, we need much more careful study of the capacities of mental defectives who are not segregated in colonies or institutions. We ought to know what percentage succeed industrially, in what kinds of occupations they are engaged, and all facts which might throw light on the causes of their success. This information should be correlated with their mental age and the training they have received. It may well be that high-grade defectives and subnormals are performing more varied types of work than they are believed by many to be capable of doing.

SPECIAL ABILITY IN NUMBER WORK

The fact that individuals with general mental defect may have unusual ability in number work has been recognized in the case of some mathematical prodigies who show great disability in all other respects. Considering the fact that the correct manipulation of the four fundamental processes, adding, subtracting, multiplying, and dividing, depends largely upon rote memory, a function often extremely good even in the feeble-minded, it is not at all surprising that even feeble-minded children may be accurate and often fairly rapid in such performances. Of course, it is quite a different story when we reach the more difficult phases of number work, which are concerned with problems in which reasoning is involved.

We need not here give instances of defectives who have learned the rudimentary aspects of number work, since this is so very common, but occasionally one meets a subnormal child who seems to have a good grasp of the operations of arithmetic. Such children are able sometimes to do so-called mental arithmetic rapidly, even though they themselves are unable to analyze the mental processes sufficiently to explain their methods.

The practical significance of special ability of this kind is quite obvious. In an institution, or outside, such facility in dealing with number combinations could be utilized. Certainly, it would be a help in all business relations and might be the main consideration in vocational guidance of individuals so gifted. There is every reason to suppose that, given certain other qualities, such as honesty and trustworthiness, a defective with this special ability might be qualified for a position as cashier.

Case 40. Martin T., 16 years old, had attended school from his sixth year, but had only reached the fifth grade when he withdrew at fourteen years. His record was poor, he had been a truant, and had several times repeated his grades.

The psychological examination showed very plainly the innate mental weakness of the boy and equally as significantly the special ability, which had apparently never been recognized, or at least put to any use. The boy did so poorly on various tests that he had to be regarded as undoubtedly subnormal in general; on the Binet scale his final score stood as several tests beyond the level for ten years. Reasoning powers, except as required in arithmetic, were markedly defective. Replies to common-sense questions, such as are given in the Binet tests, were very stupid, showing poor powers of comprehension and apperception. This was corroborated by the results on a number of different tests. He did very poorly on tests for mental analysis, showed poor control of verbal associations, and very poor powers of motor control. Memory for rote material was somewhat better, as was his ability to handle simple concrete material. Results on these latter tests were not unusual in any way, but were good in comparison with the problems involving comprehension of abstractions.

His school work was poor on the whole. He was unable to spell correctly even fairly simple words; indeed, when asked to write from dictation "The printer made some cards", the only word written correctly was "the." He read a third-grade passage haltingly, showing unfamiliarity with words in common use. But when number work was done some very interesting results were found. The boy had evidently never learned thoroughly the processes as such. He did not know how to do a problem in long division, and multiplying by two numbers he did as follows: First, he obtained the product of the first number correctly, then multiplied this product by the second number instead of using the multiplicand. Thus, while he knew the combinations of the multiplication tables, he did not know the method of handling a two-place multiplier. His lack of knowledge in regard to the proper solution of such numerical operations was probably due to a lack of training, for the boy had been truant much.

On all number work performed orally, — so-called "mental arithmetic", — the boy did extremely well. To our very great surprise he was quick in the solving of arithmetical problems. He very promptly told us the change that would be left if he had $2.00 and spent $1.47. Given the cost of one article he promptly gave the correct answer as to the cost of any multiple of this, or conversely, if told the price of a dozen oranges, for example, he readily gave the cost of any portion of a dozen. He rapidly gave the correct answer to the following problem: "If you had some apples and gave away one-half and lost one-half of those left and then had four, how many must you have had at first?" For comparison with this we must remember that this boy was unable to detect the absurdity in such a statement as "Yesterday I saw a man walking on the street with his hands in his pockets swinging a cane", nor did he give what is accounted a correct reply to the common-sense question as to what he would do before undertaking an important affair, or why one should judge a person by his acts rather than by his words.

Here is a boy, then, who shows very poor judgment and powers of reasoning in regard to many simple situations of real life, and who, nevertheless, is able to deal with number combinations very rapidly. He adds and makes change without any trouble, he can reason in regard to situations involving numerical relationships, and he can carry on processes in "his head" far better than he can do anything else. One can hardly explain his lack of school knowledge and his poor ability in reading and writing altogether on the basis of his truancy, because he had been held for several periods in a school for truants, where the instruction and training is known to be good. Furthermore, his general subnormality is evidenced by his poor results on a number of tests, many of which are not dependent upon school training.

After leaving school Martin had gone to work, but was said never to be able to keep a job. He had been employed as errand boy by several different business firms, but apparently had never been interested in any work that he had tried. No physical troubles could be held accountable for his retardation or vocational failures. He was a big, strong, very well developed boy, in excellent physical condition, except for tonsils which were somewhat enlarged. He had never been seriously ill, according to the family history which we obtained from the parents.

No special training had been give him in the subject in which the boy excelled, nor had any cognizance been taken of it in the work that had been obtained for him. He had been placed, we know, through an agency in several different positions, but without any regard to his general stupidity or his special ability. Whether any practical measures taking into account his gift for manipulation of numbers could have been undertaken, is open to discussion. When the boy was studied by us he had already been long delinquent and was not altogether trustworthy, so that he was unfitted for handling money. He had been engaged in several stealing affairs, was fond of gambling, and had once been in a burglary. To what extent his mentality was a direct factor in his misconduct we cannot be sure, but it probably had much relationship to his early truancy, which, as we know, so often leads to more serious misdeeds.

In any case, his ability for handling numbers and number relationships might well have been used to advantage; perhaps with training the boy might have been more interested in some clerical work than in the positions that had been procured for him without regard to his special ability and disabilities.

SPECIAL ABILITY FOR LANGUAGE

Some mental defectives have special ability for language, exhibited not only by the acquirement of a remarkably good vocabulary, but also by the effective and often dramatic use of words. We have known subnormal and even rather low grade feeble-minded individuals who, without special training, have shown facility in the use of several languages. The practical bearings of this talent are extremely important. Because lay verdicts regarding mental ability are based largely upon impressions gained through conversation, such people are usually accounted quite normal and even bright. It is generally felt that if a person is able to talk coherently and well, he must, perforce, be intelligent.

This type of special ability has been discussed at length by Healy in his textbook. He shows the misconceptions that often arise in the courtroom concerning the mentality of the mentally defective verbalist, as well as the serious consequences to which such faulty judgments lead. We may repeat very briefly the position taken in regard to the influence which this particular talent exerts on psychological examinations. Naturally, tests which depend upon language ability would be well performed, thus obscuring the fact that in other respects the individual may be exceedingly lacking. Since Binet tests particularly involve the use of language, this becomes a vital matter in the testing of school cases, as well as court cases, for in so many instances the Binet tests alone are relied upon for mental diagnosis. It is quite possible that this ability, together with good rote memory, would enable a child to maintain his position in the ordinary classroom for a few years before he is recognized as a defective with special ability. When reasoning and judgment are required, the defects, of course, begin to be apparent, and yet, from our own experience we know that there are cases where the individual is accounted normal by all who come into contact with him until a psychological examination reveals the truth.

The negative aspects of this problem are more striking than the positive ones, for without other abilities it is difficult to see how facility in the field of language can be practically useful; in most, if not all, positions in the social world parrot-like ability to talk well will not suffice. In consequence of their special gift, most of the defectives with special language ability whom we have seen have been socially dangerous; they have been able to impose upon all who know them and to pass among their associates as normal, even when their behavior has indicated great stupidity. Educational and vocational failures, puzzling perhaps because of this deceptive semblance of normal mentality, can be understood only when this type of special ability is appreciated in all its practical bearings.

Case 41. Wilhelmina T., 18 years old, was a girl who made an extremely favorable impression. She talked very well, expressing herself in good English. She enjoyed expressing her views of life, and for a girl of her age she had quite a philosophy, crude and immature, but fairly consistent. She had attended school for eight years, according to her parents, and had reached the sixth grade when she withdrew. Both her parents and her teachers regarded her progress as unsatisfactory, but the latter had never stated that she was below normal mentally. The girl had many advantages; her parents were intelligent, the home a very good one, earlier the family had traveled quite extensively, and later the girl had received private instruction in music and elocution.

The results of the psychological examination were surprising, because they were so little in accord with the exceedingly good impression which the girl made in conversation. It was evident that she had a special gift for language, for she did well all tests where ability to express oneself was an aid. Indeed, with the single exception of the test for psychomotor control, the only good results were achieved on the opposites test which requires control of verbal associations, on reading, and on writing sentences.

On the other hand, after noting the failures made on many comparatively simple tasks, one had little doubt of the girl's limitations. On construction tests she showed no resourcefulness; her reactions were childish, and she wished repeatedly to be allowed to stop before the expiration of the time limit. Urged to continue, she was unable to solve even the simplest test of this type. She showed no greater ability in dealing with abstractions; tests for mental representation were not only failures, but the purpose of the tests was not even grasped. The girl herself said, "I can't think of it or remember it; it's too hard." It was evident that she did not employ visual imagery as an aid; indeed we soon discovered that visual memory powers were very poor. No better success was achieved in the simple substitution test.

When the failures were analyzed it was seen that Wilhelmina was exceedingly incompetent. She not only lacked resourcefulness and planfulness, but she also did not profit by her own experiences. In reasoning and apperceptive ability she was plainly lacking; in fact, there was no single type of work done well, except language tests. Undoubtedly it was this gift for self-expression that obscured the fact of the girl's subnormality. She was stupid in general, but with special ability for language.

It was interesting to find that Wilhelmina had readily obtained several positions as salesgirl and that she was considered satisfactory in that capacity. The delinquencies in which she became involved need not be recounted here; we are interested in them only as her abilities or disabilities bear upon them. There were causative factors other than mentality, but her mental limitations formed no doubt one contributing cause; her innate defects in foresight and judgment accounted in part, at least, for the difficulties in which she became involved. What could be done constructively to aid the girl is another matter. Indeed, one could only urge that she be carefully protected, and that her general disability be recognized in order that demands which she would not be equal to meet should not be made.

Case 42.   Below is cited briefly the case of a girl who, although very definitely low-grade feeble-minded, yet was not generally recognized as such because of her ability to talk well.

Catherine L. came to this country a stranger, illiterate, untrained, but because of remarkable language ability was able to obtain and hold positions, to interest people in her behalf, and to make an extremely good impression, all on the basis of her vivacious and fluent conversation.

Catherine had been but sixteen months in this country, having come to join relatives. Her mother remained in Europe. Because of poor family circumstances she had never attended school a day in her life. She had lived in a small country town and had received no trade training, or, for that matter, training of any kind.

When we saw the girl she was able to converse fluently in English. She had quite a good vocabulary and a great deal of feeling for choice of words. She spoke dramatically, and the effectiveness of her special gift was seen in the fact that she had been able to obtain positions which, had her real defects been known, would never have been given her. Thus, she was going from door to door selling some patent appliance, having had some friend read for her the advertisement through which she had gotten her position as canvasser. She could not keep account of the money which she received in exchange for her goods, so she invented a very plausible story, asking her customers to make out a receipt which stated the amount which they had given her; then later she had others count the money which she turned over to her employers. Although so shrewd in this, her general apperceptions were poor, and she was so lacking in foresight that she soon became involved in difficulties. She was exceedingly untruthful and began stealing in very stupid ways. But so favorable was the impression which she made, that, in spite of these faults, no one interested in the girl ever realized that she was a defective. She always tried to cover her misdeeds by plausible stories and the result was that gradually she was considered to be delinquent, — never feeble-minded.

It was necessary to spend much time and to make a most careful study of this girl's mentality, because one had to take into account her lack of educational opportunities and give her the benefit of the doubt in such work as depended upon this. Bearing this point in mind, we yet were convinced at the end of our study that the girl was a mental defective. She showed very poor ability to handle concrete material; although she did remember solutions of problems when they were shown her, she herself showed absolutely no power to reason. She failed on the simplest tests for powers of analysis, showed extremely poor powers of apperception on special tests as well as in her social behavior. In spite of having handled money in her daily occupation, she had not learned to add the simplest sums nor to make simple change. In every way, then, we had evidence of her poor mental endowment.

On the other hand, we were told by those who were competent to judge that she spoke well in several languages, which she had learned through residing in different countries. Her English was unexpectedly good. We took verbatim a long conversation held with Catherine, and no one would believe it possible that a feeble-minded girl could have mastered so well a new language in the length of time that she had been in this country. There was no doubt that she had a great gift for power of expression.

We see here a very clear illustration of the dangers that this talent involves. Almost any one would have been deceived by this girl, and indeed, a great deal in the way

of monetary help had been wasted, for her innate mental
defects made it all along unlikely that she would be able
to succeed.   The sympathy and money given her might
have been much more wisely expended in helping some
one who would have profited thereby.   We ourselves recommended that this girl be committed to an institution,
for we felt that the mental and social prognosis was extremely unfavorable.

SPECIAL ABILITY FOR WORK WITH CONCRETE MATERIAL

The frequency with which special ability for working
with concrete material is found among the subnormal
and even feeble-minded has already been mentioned.
Those segregated in good institutions often profit greatly
by the very thorough training they receive along lines
that are practical and useful in the upkeep of the institution.   In the special rooms of the public schools handwork
forms the greater part of the curriculum.   A questionable
feature of this is found in the practice of training children
so largely and so long with material that will probably
not be useful after the child withdraws from school;
almost none will later weave baskets and work with raffia
and reed.   In some schools we know that training for
definite trades is given, and this would seem a wise course
to pursue.   Many of the subnormal children are fitted
only for occupations that require manual ability, and if
they have some one trade at which they are able to do well,
it must surely facilitate vocational success.

Several cases are presented to illustrate the above points,
instances being taken where the level of general intelligence is comparatively low in order to demonstrate the
marked contrast that may exist and the great social import of special abilities.

Case 43. We found here the special ability in marked contrast to general subnormality yet unrecognized until revealed by the psychological examination.

Bernard G. was 17½ years old when we were asked to see him. The psychological examination gave clear evidence of the mental traits in which this boy was particularly weak and those in which he had good ability. Rote memory was much below normal for his age, and his inability to form new associations was evident in the so-called substitution learning test, where a number is to be associated with a symbol. Powers of analysis and judgment were likewise poor. Indeed, the boy did very badly with any tests for the higher mental functions. He had learned little during his seven or eight years attendance at school; his reading was very poor, and he made numerous errors on the processes in arithmetic. Judged by the Binet scale, he was a middle-grade moron.

The significant feature, however, as far as social life was concerned, was the fact that he was successful on all types of tests which require good manual and motor ability. Construction tests were done very well and quickly, in a manner showing an appreciation of the problems and a rational method of solution; indeed, they were performed quite as well as by the ordinary normal boy of his age. Motor coördinations were equally as good.

There was nothing of any significance noted on physical examination. The boy was very well developed and well nourished; he was broad-shouldered and strong.

Home conditions were not good; the father, a hard drinking man, had frequently deserted the family and had been arrested for non-support. The mother was apparently a very good woman, and Bernard was the only one of the six living children who had caused any trouble. From the mother's point of view the main problem was that this boy did not work steadily. She claimed he had a great number of positions, but he did not keep any of them long. The boy himself said that he had held one position for a year; at that time he worked in a factory, after which he had been delivery boy for a milkman.

Earlier the boy had been much of a truant. Later he had run away from home a number of times, staying away for a period as long as six months, but, of course, his father's conduct was largely responsible for this. One of the social agencies had been assisting the family, and they wished to know what was the best thing to do for this boy.

One interesting feature in this case is the fact that though the boy had attended the public schools of a large city, he had not been examined for mentality nor been placed in a special room. He had evidently been carried on from year to year. He had received no special instruction in handwork, nor had he been prepared for any trade.

As a result of the findings on tests, it was advised that this boy should not be placed in any unselected position offered; for instance, he was not fit to be a delivery boy. His memory powers were very poor, and he needed an occupation that gave him the opportunity to use those mental capacities in which he was practically as good as the normal. He probably would have made a fairly successful worker at some trade that was not too complex. Big and strong as he was, and without evidence of any severely vicious or delinquent tendencies, there seemed little reason to believe that he would be unable to maintain himself in the community if proper work were obtained for him. Aside from the problem of eugenics involved, there certainly seemed no reason why the State should support this boy.

Case 44. This case, though so briefly studied, is cited to show the successful outcome of wise vocational adjustment, even where general intelligence is low.

Leo N., 16½ years, attended public school from his seventh to his sixteenth year. He was in the fifth grade when he left school, having been promoted without really passing after two years' trial in the third grade. The principal of the school told us he always considered that Leo was "born short." The boy had never been placed in a class for subnormal children, nor had he received any special instruction of any kind. Our examination showed conclusively that most of the time spent in school had been virtually wasted; the boy's mentality precluded the possibility of his learning by the usual school methods. He had acquired very little in any of the school branches; he did not even write his own name well. He realized his limitations, saying that he was no scholar and that he could not learn to read. However, the boy showed much dexterity in manual work; he did several tests in this field very well, proving himself to have ability to reason with concrete material and to have very good psychomotor control. This boy was tested before the present Binet series was issued or our own present tests developed, but there is no doubt that Leo would have graded as feeble-minded on everything except in handling concrete material. It is to be remembered, however, that his social apperceptive ability was good. He failed on almost every other kind of test. Especially poor was his rote memory span and his learning of the substitution or arbitrary association test, nor did he remember much better ideas which were logically connected.

We strongly urged that this boy be placed at work and taught a trade where his special abilities might come into play. This was done, and he began work in a carpenter shop. The outcome has been extremely good; some five years after first seeing the boy we learned that he has never again been delinquent, that he works steadily and saves his money, is quite contented, and able to take care of himself in every way.

SPECIAL ABILITY IN ROTE MEMORY

That the subnormal, even the low-grade feeble-minded, may have remarkably good powers of rote memory is so well known that the fact requires no lengthy discussion. Merely one example of such special ability, where there is marked contrast to other powers that are quite defective, is cited.

Case 45. James C., 11½ years old, was brought to court as a truant. He had been examined previously in another clinic, and diagnosed as defective, and placed in a class for subnormal children, but did so well in his school work there that he was removed and placed in a regular grade.

Physically James was in fair general condition. Vision was very defective in one eye and slightly defective in the other, but he wore glasses which corrected this defect. Otherwise nothing significant was found. According to our findings on the Binet scale, James was just about three years retarded. It is worth noting that he failed on those Binet tests which required either reasoning or common-sense apperceptions. Even more striking was his inability to perform the construction tests, except the simplest ones. It was quite apparent that he had poor perception of relationships of form and that he did not use any reasoning in solving problems of this type. Tests for analysis and mental representation were complete failures. His general reactions were very slow and he showed poor control of verbal associations.

In contradistinction to his failures, we found that he did very well on rote memory work. Memory span was normal for his age, and furthermore, he had learned school work of the first three grades — the only ones which he had attended — so well that he was able to make quite a good record on tests for the work of these grades. He read fluently, without mispronouncing any words in a second-grade passage, and on a third-grade passage made only one error, mispronouncing the word "Autumn." He could give a correct though somewhat meagre reproduction of what he had read. His writing was quite good, and his spelling about average for his age and grade. As for number work, he could add and subtract, and knew the simpler parts of the multiplication tables.

Because of his good powers of rote memory, by means of which he had learned the ordinary school subjects of the lower grades, he was accounted by some as being considerably brighter than wider testing showed him to be. Of course, he was retarded in school, but we must remember that he had been truant a good deal, and that for a time he had been in a room for subnormal children. Later we learned that he was committed to a school for truants, from whence came the report that though the boy had some learning ability, he could not adapt himself to the régime of the institution.

In the light of the results on a number of tests, there is no doubt that this boy was subnormal or high-grade feebleminded. Probably the time will soon come when he will be unable to maintain his position in the ordinary classroom, for we have no doubt he will fail to progress when the work becomes difficult and demands reasoning and analysis, in both of which he is so lacking.

On the basis of the results of tests, one cannot feel that the best training for this boy is the ordinary handwork, so largely taught in special classes. He does not seem to have any ability for this type of work. On the other hand, it is quite possible that his good rote memory powers, by further training, might become a valuable asset in his future career. There is no reason why such a lad could not be trained to become a fairly good clerical worker. He would never be able to keep a position of responsibility where judgment was required, but he might get on very well in routine work where little was left to his own initiative or judgment.

BORDER-LINE CASES

Sometimes it is most difficult to make a clear-cut general statement in regard to mental capacities. There are border-line cases which even after long observation and perhaps repeated psychological testing still are difficult to classify. From the standpoint of practical treatment the first necessity lies in reaching a decision as to whether such individuals require institutional care or not. Beyond the point of setting forth the fact of feeble-mindedness, that is, social incompetency, the terminology used to designate general ability quantitatively is not so important, since if the special abilities and disabilities are known, good methods of training will take these into account regardless of any classification. The same is true when we consider vocational possibilities. We must remember that specialized defects of certain types may influence a number of tests and will lead to erroneous final judgment if not known as such. Thus, language disability is often such a handicap in the Binet scale that an individual otherwise normal may grade, according to this system, as feeble minded.

Case 46. To illustrate such a problem, a typical case is presented where abilities and disabilities are clearly seen, and where the mental classification is open to question.

Frederick J. was first seen when he was 13 years 9 months old. At that time he was in the third grade in school. He had been persistently truant, but engaged in no other form of deliquency. He was born in America of English speaking parents.

Physically he was in good condition, except for traces of a speech trouble which earlier had been severe. As for the mental examination, he made a very good record on the construction tests and all work with concrete material. Indeed, some of the more difficult tests, which require reasoning and quite good insight, were not very difficult for him. A striking difference was found between the auditory and visual memory fields, the former being very much better of the two. He gave a good reproduction of a passage read to him, so far as the ideas contained therein were concerned, — he omitted only one of the twelve items, — but in his account there was no adherence to verbal accuracy and little regard for logical sequence. Visual memory tests were miserable failures. It was quite apparent that the boy had exceedingly poor powers of visualization.

Perhaps this lack was a factor in the failure on tests for mental representation and analysis. On these he never succeeded even in numerous trials. After seeing a figure, he could not reproduce it from memory, nor could he recognize the various parts when the figure was analyzed. His associative processes were decidedly defective. He made many errors in giving the opposites of very simple words. He had much difficulty in forming new associations between arbitrary symbols, the record on this test being exceedingly poor.

The results on school work were quite discrepant. He did work in arithmetic out of proportion to his ability to read and write; he could add, subtract, and multiply accurately. On the other hand, he could not write anything except his own name, not even the individual letters of the alphabet; he could not read the letters when they were shown him, nor could he always recognize them, though he could say the alphabet without error. Neither could he read the simplest passage.

He failed to recognize such simple monosyllables as "am" and "in."

About two and one half years after we first saw Frederick, we had occasion to study him once more. At that time we found that his disabilities were as striking as previously. He showed much difficulty in the correct use of language and was still exceedingly defective in visual memory powers. He told us that he had made one more grade in school, having finished the fourth when he withdrew at fourteen years. In the intervening years the boy had gained practically nothing in either reading or writing; his spelling was almost unbelievably inaccurate; he could not write the name of the school which he had been attending, and it would have been impossible to have interpreted his writing without his own explanation. He still could not read, but as for number work, he performed correctly the three of the fundamental processes which he had been taught, namely, addition, subtraction and multiplication.

In view of the fact that this boy shows on psychological tests that he has certain innate defects, it is difficult to know whether he should be regarded as an out-and-out feeble-minded, or whether in the light of his good ability along certain lines it would not be practically more helpful to consider him a case of specialized defects. According to the Binet scales he grades through ten years, his failures being entirely on language tests and the one for visual memory. Of course, his disabilities are quite extensive. Without doubt he is extremely poor in visual powers and likewise in the field of language. Perhaps these two weaknesses will account for his poor records on association tests and form the basis of his inability to learn reading, writing, and spelling; but on the other hand it might be argued that his ability to learn arithmetic and to make ordinary computations, as well as his capabilities along motor lines, are simply special capacities not at all incompatible with feeble-mindedness. One could present quite good arguments for either diagnosis.

Practically, however, as above stated, it does not much matter if one reaches the conclusion that the boy is not a fit subject for an institution. We know, at least, that certain types of work are well-nigh impossible for him to learn, and that he will probably always be unsuited for certain occupations. On the other hand, he should have training along industrial lines and then later engage in some definite trade. Whether he could ever gain even moderate facility in the handling of language and learn to read and write, is a doubtful matter, since his disabilities are pretty widespread. We do not know that any emphasis was placed upon phonetic drill in his schooling so that the boy could benefit by his good auditory powers, or that any methods were ever used adapted to his particular problem. One interesting fact which always stood in the way of proper training with this lad was the father's attitude; he said he did not want the boy to use tools, he wanted him to be "educated."

CHAPTER X

GENERAL CONCLUSIONS

IT is not the author's purpose to offer any specific devices guaranteed to overcome defects or to develop abilities. Since each individual problem-case would seem to require intelligent consideration on the basis of all data that can be gathered concerning it, it naturally follows that no general formulæ for treatment can be given, no dogmatic statements made in regard to general constructive measures. Rather, we would reiterate a trite and perhaps commonplace observation that the human mind is wonderfully complex, that, in consequence, capacities frequently can be determined only by painstaking investigation and thoughtful consideration of all that goes to make the given results on tests.

The first principle of progress towards the goal of developing each individual in relation to his potentialities is recognition of the actual need for individual adjustment. To realize that such a problem exists, to be able to formulate it clearly in one's own mind, to see its significance and its relation to life, is the first step toward its solution. It has been the purpose in the preceding chapters to present types of abilities and disabilities that require special consideration, as well as to prove the practical importance of directing efforts in accordance with these mental characteristics.

We must view critically the present means for meeting the situation. Ungraded classes, "floating teachers", junior and senior high schools and other administrative measures, advancement in school by subjects rather than by grades, are all helpful, but inadequate. Courses in household and practical arts, commercial, industrial, and agricultural training, offer greater scope for adapting education to individual capacities and interests than was possible in the past, but these, too, are not enough. More fundamental than all of these, because offering the basis of the wise and rational use of all special training, is the need for educational diagnosis. Before undertaking treatment the ailment must be known; the cause of the trouble must be determined before steps can be taken looking toward effective remedy. This is as true of mental peculiarity as of physical troubles, and it applies in educational and vocational life as truly as in any other field.

Of course we must appreciate the complexities inherent in any effort to study an individual's mental characteristics, and while realizing the folly of minimizing the difficulties and limitations, we should not lose sight of the many important and helpful facts that can be learned. At present there are many gaps in the knowledge required for a scientific study of human beings; we cannot always distinguish between mental traits; we do not know with surety where one process ends and another begins, or how one is related to another. We do not know the best age at which to study individuals in order to determine the facts which should modify education. Mental tests in their present stage of development cannot answer all our problems.

This is, however, no reason why we should not make use of such means of reaching helpful conclusions as are now available. Even though subtle distinctions cannot be made and minute individual differences discriminated, we may find many illuminating suggestions in special instances of failures and successes. There is little value in the effort to read into results of tests more than they are known to reveal, to make on such a basis generalizations that are only assumptions not open to proof. It is wiser to confess frankly that correlations between mental processes involved in definite tests and complex activities, educational and vocational, are not yet established. But this does not lessen a whit the value of findings which indicate peculiarities in individual mental functioning. It is the part of wisdom to discover all one can of the characteristic mental traits of individuals and to guide practical procedure in the light of these findings.

Many practically valuable diagnoses may be made if we are aware of the individual differences that exist and are intelligent enough to interpret reactions that indicate need for special adaptations. Such study of mental make-up as has been indicated in the chapter on Mental Diagnosis can be undertaken by those trained for the task. In the chapter on Differential Diagnosis is discussed the care which must be exercised before final conclusions are reached. If the examination is thorough and made under favorable conditions, psychological tests, in spite of all possible criticisms, illuminate many a situation and give an insight into traits that are fundamental for training and for vocational life.

We know, for instance, of a boy now 14 years old whose entire school career has undoubtedly been greatly modified for the better because his intelligent parents understood better than his teachers the harm that was resulting from the use of methods not adapted to his defective functioning in certain mental processes. It was early recognized that the boy had poor auditory powers and exceptionally good visual powers. When five years old he drew a very good representation of the façade of an ancient university building he had seen, and at seven made a most complicated drawing of a quadruple expansion waterworks engine. Though a great effort was made from the time he was a year or so old to teach him Mother-Goose rhymes and other couplets, he never recited correctly the simplest verse until he was six years old; nor has he ever been able to carry a tune correctly or sing a song, in spite of intensive and oft repeated attempts to teach him simple music. It is interesting to note, for instance, that "America" has been sung and played to him hundreds of times and even been played by him without his acquiring the ability to sing it.

At five years of age this boy was sent to a fine private school where the teaching in the first grades was largely oral. When in the third grade he was placed in a subclass for backward children because he was so retarded in number work. Though the boy made no progress in music nor in memorizing verses, this was not interpreted as of any significance, nor was any effort made to utilize his good visual powers in place of his defective powers of audition. When, however, his parents were told (by an unusually competent teacher) that the boy was not learning arithmetic and was probably defective in this type of work, they themselves began to teach him by visual presentations. In two weeks he had not only mastered the work assigned the grade, but led his class. In the next two years, acquiring the power to learn by visualization, he accomplished the ordinary work of four school grades. Now, at fourteen, through extensive compensations, little difficulty arises; he transposes, probably often unconsciously, many auditory percepts into visual form. His own introspections, as well as his method of studying, show very conclusively that visual means are employed whenever possible. His powers of perceiving logical relationships are extremely good, and these, together with his quite unusual visual gifts, enable him to maintain class standings considerably in advance of his years. It is interesting that even now his greatest disability is in regard to language; in spite of all the advantages derived from the best of environmental conditions, the boy shows poor feeling in the use of English. In dealing with foreign languages there is great aptness displayed in learning the structural form, but quite a little trouble with achieving an idiomatic translation. It is evident that in this field he is hardly at all aided by sound.

From such concrete examples of what must be frequently occurring in school life we can draw several practical conclusions. One important point to emphasize is that our experience has shown us in large measure that unfortunately the present tendency in mental and educational diagnosis is to emphasize only defects and disabilities, to grade the child down, rather than up. Little or no effort is made to discover if there are any gifts or unusual abilities that might offer hope for useful development. In contrast to this we must insist that if there is any desire to attain the greatest measure of success and usefulness, the good as well as the bad must be regarded, the positive as well as the negative aspects, the potentialities as well as the disabilities.

What can be done to compensate for or to minimize defect can only be determined on the basis of the special conditions that exist in each individual case. In general the balance should be preserved between reasonable expenditure of time and energy and the value of the results that we may hope to achieve. To make no attempt to improve the defective condition will surely not be wise; what definite steps shall be undertaken and how long they shall be continued, depends in each case upon the original diagnosis and upon the improvement that follows definite training of various types. The possibilities or the limitations can be learned only through experimental endeavors with each individual. If the defect is the direct cause of failure in a subject that can be learned in some other way, common sense alone would urge that methods be used based on the powers that would give mastery of the subject. After all, attainment of such mastery is the end, and means or methods used are valuable in direct proportion to the measure of success in achieving the end.

Analysis of the mental processes which are elements in activities for which defect exists would seem to offer the greatest hope of rationally attacking the problems of specialized incapacity. We have attempted to make such analysis for school subjects in the case of language and number work. As experimentation progresses, much greater knowledge will, no doubt, be gained concerning the psychology of these and other complex activities as well as of the separate mental processes. This knowledge can then be applied in the solving of such problems as those of educational and vocational adjustments.

The exact degree to which defective powers can be improved is not definitely known, no matter whether the defect concerns perception, memory, association, speed of reactions, or any other phase of mental life. But definite training and practice are so generally effective — many experimental studies of the learning process also prove the fact — that it seems only fair to conclude that even where powers are exceedingly low they can be vastly increased by intensive training.

To what extent visual, auditory, motor, or other types of presentation should be stressed in education can be determined only in the light of what is learned concerning the abilities and disabilities in each of these fields. If there is a defect in any one of these aspects of mental life, devices should be found for developing the defective power in as far as this is possible, while compensating powers should be utilized as well. The same general principle applies to the relative emphasis to be placed on either memory or reasoning, wherever the problem is that of habituation versus rationalization.

Where concepts are lacking, actual experience with the concrete should precede further efforts to master abstractions. The step from the concrete to the abstract is often difficult for the child to make; in consequence it is frequently necessary to help him in making this transition. Specific devices will suggest themselves to every skillful teacher, once she is aware of the problem.[1]

There is less doubt about the procedure advisable for the utilization of special abilities. Surely, capacities that are found to exist should be trained intensively; they should be made to compensate for any other lack, in so far as this is possible. In them lies the greatest hope for the individual's future, not only from the standpoint of later vocational and industrial life, but also for the development of wholesome interests and moral welfare.

At what age the study of the mental processes, through testing and other means, should be undertaken can only be answered in general terms. For several reasons, we believe that it should be begun as soon as possible

---

[1] Unfortunately, at the present time there is no standard work on the devices which may be utilized for the training of special abilities and disabilities. Here and there, widely scattered in the literature of special subjects, there may be found treatment of particular points. One may consult with most promise of help the good bibliographies of William Stern ("Differentielle Psychologie." Leipzig, 1911) and Ernst Meumann ("Vorlesungen zur Einführung in die Experimentelle Pädagogik." 1914). In the American journals of education and psychology there are many articles that contain suggestions and hints. Of course, there are volumes on methods of teaching, both general and special, but none based on anything more than the main laws of mental life, laws which are applicable to all activities rather than to the peculiarities of special cases. In spite of much experimentation, little has been written concerning the training of the separate mental processes other than by practice.

after there is reason to believe that the individual presents a problem. Here, as elsewhere, one should not be needlessly anxious, remembering that some children learn slowly, and that frequently some time elapses before the child adjusts himself to any new conditions of school life. When failure continues after a short period of training and effort, psychological study of the mental life should be made.

The first and most obvious advantage of early investigation is the saving of time that would otherwise be wasted. The second is the prevention of discouragement and loss of interest. With the consciousness of failure there is, all too frequently, emotional disturbance leading to the development of a bad attitude, either towards the difficult subject or towards school in general. Frequently the child is subjected to teasing by his comrades, or to scolding by his teachers; sometimes friction arises at home as well as at school, and as a consequence of all these irritations, anti-social grudges are formed. Because of these conditions, leading to lack of self-confidence and sometimes to excessive mental disturbances, we find that it is often extremely difficult to induce the older child or adolescent to make any efforts under systematic guidance to overcome the defects. Again and again we have seen that in spite of desire to master the difficulty, emotions may be stronger than ambition.

One interesting discovery, mentioned several times incidentally in our case-histories, is the fact that occasionally the individual, as he grows older, realizes the cause of his failure and through his own effort, frequently clumsy, accomplishes more than years of school training had achieved. Because of this truth, we would urge that the teacher and vocational guide adopt the attitude of the scientist. If, for example, the teacher saw in each unusual child a particular problem to be solved, if reactions were viewed in the light of their significance for the solution of that problem, teaching would become vitalized. In the schoolroom and in the shop, valuable data could be gathered, various hypotheses tested, and experimental pedagogy evolved. The school, through the attitude of its teachers, could become an experimental station, — and experimental stations in connection with education are one of our most urgent needs.

Indeed, it is only through coöperation of parent, teacher, vocational guide, and even employer with the clinical psychologist that headway can be made. The clinician can offer a prognosis and recommendations for practical procedure; but the truth of the prognosis and the value of the recommendations can be determined only by surveying them in the light of the results that follow directed efforts. Analysis of successes and failures in the individual case is the only possible means of ultimately determining the correctness of a diagnosis and the efficacy of methods of treatment. And such critical evaluation, it may be added, is one essential requirement, needed almost more than anything else, for further development and growth of the science of clinical psychology.

Scientific study of human reactions is in its infancy. With the further development of mental tests, with greater ability to interpret test results, with more knowledge of the correlations that exist between different mental functions, as well as between these and educational and vocational pursuits, we may hope for vastly greater understanding of the varied problems of mental disabilities and for wiser utilization of special abilities.

APPENDIX

To aid in interpreting the summaries of case-studies cited below, a brief description is here given of the tests used, which include the Binet-Simon scale, series of 1911 unless otherwise stated; the Healy-Fernald tests, detailed description of which can be found in Psychological Monograph Number 54. To these are added a considerable number of other tests described in many different books and journals. Other measuring scales are sometimes used, especially the Terman scale; frequently the latter is employed as an alternative for retesting when the Binet scale has been previously used. Most of the cases reported were studied before the publication of the Yerkes-Bridges scale. The main tests include: —

Introductory Test: — This is a combination of the form board with the picture puzzle. The seven pieces are quite dissimilar in shape and have distinctive parts of the picture printed on them, two are nearly interchangeable, and two are right triangles which fit into an equilateral triangle. These last two give a good opportunity for studying the subject's ability to profit by trial and error.

Construction Test I: — This is a wooden frame into which five pieces are to be fitted. While there are a number of possible positions into which the various pieces can be put there is only one correct position for each piece, although any four of them can be placed in a number of ways. This test involves the subject's perception of space relationships and also shows his planfulness and ability to profit by past trials.

229

Construction Test II: — This involves the same mental elements as the first construction test. It is, however, more complex, as there are many more alternative moves.

The Puzzle Box: — The purpose of this test is to bring out abilities or defects in manipulative power and the ability to analyze a slightly complicated concrete ,situation. The box is fastened by a series of strings passed over posts which can be unfastened only in a certain sequence. As one side of the box is glass, the entire arrangement can be seen.

Cross Line Test I: — The investigator draws a large X on a sheet of paper in front of the subject, calling attention to the fact that the figure is made up of four parts. These are then numbered, the order in which the numbers are placed with regard to the figure being emphasized and after the subject has had ample chance to look at the model, it is turned over. The different angles are drawn one by one and the subject is asked to tell what number belongs in each. If he fails he is allowed to draw and number the figure himself and try again. This and the two tests following involve the power of mental representation of the model, together with the ability to analyze it into its parts and recall the numbers corresponding to the parts.

Cross Line Test II: — The procedure is the same as the above except that the figure is the one used by children in the game of " Tit-tat-to ", and is made up of nine parts.

Code Test: — By combination of the two cross line tests a complete alphabetical code can be arranged. After the subject has studied it, it is turned over, and he is given a sentence to write in the code. Because of the greater number of parts to be worked out from the subject's recollection of the general scheme, this test indicates ability to control mental processes as well as ability to grasp the idea of a code.

Pictorial Completion Test : — This test is a picture representing ten activities from which ten squares of equal size have been cut out so that on each piece is a part essential to the meaning of the whole. There are forty more pieces on which are drawn objects that do not logically complete the picture. The subject is told to insert the pieces that " make the best sense." The test indicates the subject's power of apperception with this type of material.

The Ebbinghaus Completion Test : — This is the mutilated text test where omitted words are to be supplied. The Trabue scales have been used since their publication.

Arbitrary Association or Substitution Test: — This test shows the ability of the subject to form associations between a set of symbols and numerals.

Tests of Memory for Logical Material : — Two passages, one to test auditory verbal and the other to test visual verbal memory are used.

Tests for Memory Span : — Numerals are presented auditorily and visually until the point is reached at which the subject makes an error. Sentences containing an increasing number of syllables are also used.

Tests for Visual Memory : — The usual Binet visual test is supplemented by a number of other tests, including several similar in character.

Tests for Remote Memory : — Reproduction of tests given at an earlier date, including not only memory passages, but tests for remembrance of form, events, etc.

Tapping Test : — In this test for psychomotor control the subject inserts a dot as rapidly as possible in half inch squares without touching the lines or missing the squares.

Tests for Controlled Association: — The subject is given a word to which he is to reply by a word bearing an assigned relationship to the stimulus word; the relationship may be that of opposite, genus-species, agent-object, mixed relationship, etc. The lists standardized by Woodworth and Wells are used ; the time reaction for each word is recorded.

Kraepelin Addition and Subtraction Tests : — These are the well known continuous addition and subtraction tests used to gauge mental control.

Aussage Test : — The butcher-shop picture is exposed for ten seconds, after which the subject gives a free account of what he has seen, followed by answers to direct questions.

Instruction Box : — Six steps are necessary to open a box. These steps are shown the subject, who then is to follow the directions given. The errors made and the number of trials required to open the box are recorded.

Analogies Test : — We use the test as given in the Yerkes-Bridges, Terman, and other scales. The subject is to insert in each of five sentences a word bearing the same relationship to another given word as is shown in the first half of the sentence, *e.g.* " Oyster is to shell as banana is to —."

Tests for Arithmetical Reasoning : — We use the Terman test, placed at the 15-year level, and many other problems, according to age and school experience of the subject.

Terman Ball and Field Test : — The problem is to devise the best and most economical method of finding a ball lost in a circular field of high grass.

Link Chain Test : — Five pieces of chain, each consisting of three links, are to be joined by making not more than three cuttings.

Stenquist Test for Mechanical Ability : — A number of models are placed before the subject together with the parts with which he can make the different objects by copying from the models.

Woodworth-Wells Directions Tests : — The subject follows directions given in printed form. Several sets are used ; in some the directions to be followed are more difficult than in others.

Tests for Visual Perception Plus Attention : — The well known cancellation test.

Questionnaire Tests for Ordinary Information.

Tests for Common-sense Adaptations : — These include telling time, handling money, environmental orientation, etc.

Still other tests are used in special cases for purposes of differential diagnosis. For example : — The Kent-Rosanoff Test; repetition of phrases requiring good auditory discrimination ; drawing floor plans ; Yerkes Multiple-Choice test ; some of the Rossolimo tests, particularly giving backwards the months of the year and obeying several commands; Knox Cube test, etc.

TEST RECORDS OF CASES GIVEN IN THE TEXT

Case 1. EDITH N. 12 years, 3 months.

Binet grade: 9⅔ years. Failures: 8 years (4); 9 years (1); 10 years (3) and (4). **Introductory Test:** 3′ 57″, of which 2′ 43″ were spent on the triangles. **Construction Test I:** Failure. **School Work:** Writes from dictation " I had sone money and drop in river." **Arithmetic:** Adds simple combinations, *e.g.* 7 + 8 = 15; fails to add four 3-place numerals.

Second Testing 13 months later:

Binet grade: Through 12 years. **Introductory Test:** 2′ 5″, of which 1′ 15″ were spent on the triangles. **Construction Test I:** 2′ 1″, 22 moves. **Construction Test II:** 1′ 15″, 17 moves. **Cross Line Test I:** Correct third trial. **Pictorial Completion Test:** 3′ 32″, 2 illogical errors. **Easy Opposites Test:** No errors or failures, average time 1.5″. **Auditory Memory Span:** 6 numerals correct. **School Work:** Writes from dictation " The cat ran away." " The grirl gos to scholl." Reading 3rd-grade passage. Errors made on longer words, such as " autumn ", " frightened ", " opening." Reproduction is meager but correct. Still adds correctly 2 numbers orally, but fails on 2-column addition. Cannot subtract. Knows only simplest combinations of the multiplication table.

Case 2. ADAM F. 9 years.

Binet: 6- and 7-year tests all correct; 8-year tests correct, except (4); 9-year tests, 1, 3, and 5 correct; fails (2) and (4). Cannot read or do number work.

Case 3. ROLAND M. 12 years, 9 months.

Binet : Passes all the 12-year tests correctly. Fails visual test of the 10-year group. (Notably good results achieved on many of these tests.) **Introductory Test :** 2′ 30″. **Pictorial Completion Test :** 4′ 3″, no errors. (Time reaction lengthened by visual defect.) **School Work :** Writes from

dictation " The printer made some cards." Arithmetic :
Adds and subtracts ; knows simple number combinations.
Reads 5th-grade passage somewhat slowly owing to difficulty
in seeing ; gives good reproduction. Recites stanzas from
poems of Longfellow.

Case 4. CAROLINE J. 14 years, 3 months.
Construction Test II : Complete failure. Cross Line Test
I : Correct at first trial. Cross Line Test II : Utter failure.
(Could do nothing more at this time because of the girl's
attitude ; she cried and made a scene. Diagnosis had to be
left in abeyance.)
Second Testing one year later :
Binet : Through 10 years. (But not all of the Binet tests
were given on account of the girl's attitude.) Construction
Test I : 17", 6 moves ; good performance. Construction
Test II : 2' 14", 19 moves ; also a good result. Cross Line
Test I : Correct first trial. Cross Line Test II : Correct at
third trial ; not a good performance. Pictorial Completion
Test : 2' 52" ; 2 errors, 1 logical and 1 illogical. Tapping
Test : 87 and 90 squares respectively on first and second
trial ; 1 error in each ; good performance. Memory for
Logical Material — visual verbal presentation : Maintained
that she could not remember at all the passage which she
read ; said it was all gone from her after she had given the
first item. Memory for Logical Material — auditory verbal
presentation : 8 items given, but these were poorly phrased
although in logical sequence ; altogether a distinctly poor
result. Auditory Memory Span : only 5 numerals correct.
Opposites Test : (Association for 20 easy opposites) 3 failures,
2 errors ; average time 3". Kraepelin Subtraction Test :
Very poor result on several trials, many errors made. Aussage : Very meager account given in free recital, only 7
items ; on cross-examination 22 items given, but 8 of these
were incorrect. However, only one out of seven suggestions
offered was accepted. School Work : Reading : Equivalent
of 5th-grade passage ; fluent, but without much expression ;
only the harder words not known. Writing and Spelling :

Writes neatly and rapidly; fairly good hand. Arithmetic: Long division done with much erasing ; 1 error.

Third Testing eighteen months later :

Binet grade : Through all of the 10 and 12-year tests except (3) of the 12-year set. **Cross Line Test II** : Correct at first trial. **Pictorial Completion Test** : 1′ 50″ ; 3 errors, 2 illogical. **Tapping Test** : 95 and 93 squares respectively on first and second trial ; 1 and 2 errors respectively. **Opposites Test** : (Another set of easy opposites) 3 errors, 2 failures ; average time 2.1″. **Kraepelin Subtraction Tests** : Subtracting 3 from 44, all correct, 33″ ; subtracting 4 from 51, 4 errors, 1′ 8″.

Case 5. JASPER B. 13 years, 7 months.

Binet : The 9 and 10-year tests correct ; 12-year tests, 1 and 3 correct, 2, 4, and 5 failures. **Construction Test I** : 6″, 6 moves. **Construction Test II** : 1′, 15 moves. **Cross Line Test I** : correct second trial. **Cross Line Test II** : correct first trial. **Pictorial Completion Test** : 2′ 18″, 5 errors, 3 illogical. **Continuous Subtraction Test** : 4 from 51, 1′, 1 error. **School Work** : Writes "The boy go to school." Arithmetic : adds, subtracts, and multiplies correctly. Reads 3rd-grade passage fairly well ; gives meager but correct reproduction.

Case 6. JEROME B. 16 years.

First Testing:

No psychological tests given because school work was done exceptionally well. Boy is in 8th grade. Solves correctly examples in adding, subtracting and multiplying fractions. Solves by ingenious method examples in interest. Has very good school record as regards ability.

Second Testing two years, nine months later at correctional institution.

Binet grade : 10⅕ years. 8-year tests correct except (5) ; 9-year tests all correct ; 10-year tests, 3, 4, and 5 correct, 1 and 2 failures. 12-year tests, 1, 3, and 5 correct, 2 and 5 failures; 15-year tests, 2 correct, 1, 3, and 5 failures.

Construction Test I: 52″, 20 moves. **Substitution Test:** no errors. **Hard Directions Test:** 2 errors. **School Work:** Arithmetic, still solves examples in fractions and interest correctly.

Third Testing 3 months after last testing:

Binet : through the 12-year tests and three additional tests correct. All 10-year tests correct ; 12-year tests correct except (1) ; all 15-year tests except (3). (Very good results in many instances ; thus, gave 60 words in 25″ ; interpretation of pictures very good.) **Auditory Memory Span :** 8 numerals correct. **Easy Opposites Test :** 1 error, average time 1.3″. Reads difficult advertisement correctly and fluently ; gives good reproduction.

Case 7. WILLARD Z. 15½ years old.

Binet : All the 10 and 12-year tests correct ; well and readily done. **Construction Test I :** 22″, 7 moves ; very good result. **Construction Test II :** 53″, 11 moves ; extremely good result. **Cross Line Test I :** Correct first trial. **Cross Line Test II :** Failure on fourth trial. **Pictorial Completion Test :** 2′ 26″ ; 1 logical error. **Auditory Memory Span :** Only 4 numerals correct. Fails on 5 numerals in each of four trials. **Visual Memory Span :** 7 numerals correct ; fails on 8 numerals in each of three trials. **School Work :** Writes from dictation "The printer made some cards." Reading : 5th-grade passage, fluent, good expression, and reproduction correct. Arithmetic : (written work) : Absolute failure on addition of four 3-place numerals. Subtraction, multiplication and division failures. (Oral) : Fails on problems such as the following : $7 + 8 + 3 \times 2$. Says $7 + 4 = 14$, or 13, or 12. Subtracts correctly 7 from 50 but says $100 - 8 = 90$. Simple multiplication combinations, such as 8×5 correct ; but many others incorrect, *e.g.* $9 \times 9 = 63$; $7 \times 7 = 42$. Adds change correctly, but even with money in his hand cannot make change. $\$1.00 - 87 ¢ = 27 ¢$; $\$2.00 - \$1.37 = 59 ¢$. Says at 48 ¢ a dozen 5 oranges cost 26 ¢.

Second Testing 3 months later :

Cross Line Test II : Correct first trial. **Easy Opposites Test** : 1 error, no failures ; average time 1.7″. **Arbitrary Association Test** : no errors. **Woodworth-Wells Easy Directions Test** : (first set) 1′ 55″, 2 errors ; (second set) 1′ 32″, no errors. **Hard Directions Test** : 2′ 50″, 4 errors. **Auditory Memory Span** : 4 numerals correct but only once in three trials. **Memory for Logical Material—visual verbal presentation** : 15 of 20 items in correct logical sequence. **Memory for Logical Material — auditory verbal presentation** : 10 of 12 items ; logical sequence incorrect and little verbal accuracy ; ideas, however, correct. **School Work** : Reading difficult "Want Ad", reproduction correct except for numbers; cannot remember the number of building and room at which to apply. **Arithmetic** : Fails again on addition, subtraction, multiplication, and long division, although he has been attending night school. Fails again to make change, *e.g.* $1.00 − 87 ¢, and becomes utterly confused ; cannot make the change with money before him. Fails to return the change, *e.g.* 50 ¢ − 35 ¢. Gives change correctly only when multiples of 5 are required. Cannot tell the cost of ⅔ of a dozen when 1 dozen cost 24 ¢ ; fails on other similar problems.

Case 8. ALFRED T. 16½ years old.

Introductory Test : 2′ 35″, no repetitions of errors. **Construction Test I** : 13″, 6 moves ; remarkably good result. **Construction Test II** : 50″, 11 moves (the smallest possible number), also notably good result. **Puzzle Box** : 1′ 20″ ; very rapid perception of correct solution. **Tapping Test** : 74 and 75 squares, respectively, at first and second trials; no errors. **Instruction Box** : Done correctly third trial (compare this rather poor result with good record on Puzzle Box). **Cross Line Test I** : Correct at third trial. **Cross Line Test II** : Correct first trial. **Arbitrary Association Test** : 4 errors ; very poor result. **Visual Memory — reproduction of Binet geometric figures** : Result very good. **Memory for Logical Material — visual verbal presentation** : 17 of 20 items given in correct logical sequence. **Memory for Logical Material — auditory verbal presentation** : 8 of 12 items given in correct sequence, inaccuracies in minor details. **Easy Opposites Test** : 2 failures ; 2 errors ; average time 3.2." **School Work** : Writes from dictation " The printer naid some cards." Reading : 5th-grade passage, reads " part " for " party ", " man " for " men ", " walk " for "work ", mispronunciation, probably due to carelessness. Arithmetic : Adding five 3-place numerals, 1 error ; very slowly done. Has no conception of solution of simple problem in interest, although has had months of training in business course.

Case 9. MARY L. 10 years, 9 months.

Binet grade : 9⅗ years. Failures : 9-year (1) ; 10-year, (2). **Construction Test I** : 1' 35", 12 moves. **Pictorial Completion Test** : 3' 34", 1 logical error. **Auditory Memory Span**: 5 numerals correct. **School Work** : Writes from dictation " I am going to school Tuesday ", and sentences of about equal difficulty. Reading : 3rd-grade passage, she fails on a few of the longer words, but reads fluently and with good expression. Arithmetic : adds simple number combinations slowly, *e.g.*, $6 + 5 + 9 = 20$; fails on subtraction and multiplication.

Second Testing 8 months later.

Binet grade : through 10 years and 3 of the 12-year tests. **Construction Test II** : 2' 33", 17 moves. **Cross Line Test I**: correct first trial. **Cross Line Test II** : correct 4th trial, but only very slowly and with considerable effort. **Arbitrary Association Test** : no errors. **Auditory Memory Span** : 5 numerals correct. **School Work** : Arithmetic (written) : adds four 3-place numerals correctly. Cannot subtract, for example, says $50 - 42 = 10$; says $7 - 7 = 7$. (Oral) Some combinations of multiplication table correct and others failures, *e.g.*, $4 \times 3 = 12$; $4 \times 8 = 32$, but $4 \times 6 = 22$. Fails to give correct answer to, $25¢ - 8¢ = ?$; $25¢ - 4¢ = ?$; says $10¢ - 6¢ = 4¢$. With actual change cannot add 50¢ and 25¢, nor solve $50¢ - 42¢$. Given a quarter and asked to return the change after 18¢ is spent, shows much difficulty in mental representation of the problem. Counts the 18¢ in change and then tries to find what is needed to make up the 25 ¢, but since it cannot be done with the change before her, fails to solve the problem.

Case 10. JOHN T. 14 years, 10 months.

Binet grade : Through the 12-year tests, and passes 1, 2, and 5 of the 15-year tests. **Construction Test I** : 1′ 35″, 16 moves. **Construction Test II** : 1′ 2″, 13 moves. **Cross Line Test I** : Correct on first trial. **Cross Line Test II** : Correct on second trial. **Pictorial Completion Test** : 2′ 27″, 1 logical error. **School Work** : Writes from dictation " The printer made some cards." 5th-grade passage read fluently and reproduction good. Arithmetic (written work) : fails to add four 3-place numerals ; cannot subtract, multiply, or divide. (Oral) : Gives correctly the combinations of the multiplication table. Says 5 apples plus 7 apples equal 12 ; 8 apples plus 5 apples equal 15 ; says present year is 1915 and that he is 14 years old and therefore was born in 1902. 2 dimes equal 20 cents ; 2 nickels equal 10 cents ; 2 dimes, 2 nickels and 2 pennies equal 95 cents ; a quarter and a nickel make 35 cents ; 50 cents minus 35 cents equals? (failure) ; a half dollar and a quarter makes $1.25. (All problems done with change before him.) If a dozen cost 24 cents 5 cost? (failure). How many inches on the 4 sides of a 2-inch square? After 40 seconds says he does not know (restates the problem correctly).

Case 11. HENRY M. 10 years, 11 months.

Introductory Test : 1′ ; perceptions very good, no trial and error used ; remarkably well done. **Construction Test I** : 20″, 5 moves ; smallest number possible. **Construction Test II** : 30″, 11 moves ; also smallest number possible. **Puzzle Box** : 1′ 50″, 3 errors ; planful procedure. **Instruction Box** : 40″ ; correct first trial ; rapidly and understandingly done. **Tapping Test** : 63 and 70 squares on first and second trial respectively, 1 and 2 errors. **Pictorial Completion Test** : 1′ 45″, no errors. **Cross Line Test I** : Correct on first trial. **Cross Line Test II** : Correct on first trial. **Visual Memory Test — reproduction of Binet figures** :

Well done. **Auditory Memory Span :** 6 numerals correct. **Memory for Logical Material** — visual verbal presentation : 12 of 20 items; 1 change in logical sequence. **Memory for Logical Material** — auditory verbal presentation : 11 of 12 items correct ; correct sequence and fair verbal accuracy. **Arbitrary Association Test :** no errors ; done promptly. **School Work :** Writes from dictation, " The preuter made some cards." Arithmetic (written) : Fails to add four 4-place numerals ; fails on long division ; makes errors here in process of division and in subtraction. (Oral) : Gives the combinations of multiplication tables correctly ; says $4 \times 6 + 7 - 8 = 16$; $5 \times 7 + 6 - 8 = 15$; is able to restate problems.

Case 12. LILLIAN M. 14 years, 11 months.
Introductory Test : 38″ ; very quick perception ; no trial and error used. **Construction Test I :** 27″, 10 moves. **Construction Test II :** 40″, 11 moves. **Tapping Test :** 76 and 90 squares, first and second trial respectively ; no errors. **Cross Line Test I :** Correct on first trial. **Cross Line Test II :** Correct on first trial. **Code Test :** 2 errors. **Pictorial Completion Test :** 3′ 8″, 2 logical errors and 1 illogical error. **School Work :** Writes from dictation, " The printer made some cards." Reading : 5th-grade passage read fluently. Arithmetic (written) : Adds correctly five 4-place numerals — slowly done ; multiplication and long division failure. (Oral): Subtracting continuously 7 from 100, 1′ 32″, 10 errors.

Case 13. ARTHUR L. 17 years old.
Binet grade : Through 12-year, no errors ; tests done rapidly and well. **Construction Test I :** 3′ 21″, 42 moves. **Construction Test II :** 46″, 12 moves. **Cross Line Test II :** Correct on first trial. **Opposites Test :** No errors or failures ; average time 1.4″. **School Work :** Writes from dictation, " The printer made some cards." Reading : 5th grade well read, fair reproduction. Arithmetic (written): Fails on long division ; numerous errors in multiplication

and occasional errors in subtraction. (Oral): says $2.00 less $1.57 equals 48 cents ; at 36 cents a dozen 5 oranges cost 6½ cents. Subtracting continuously 7 from 100, 2' 12", 9 errors.

Case 14. ADOLPH J. 15 years, 8 months.

Binet grade : Through 12-year tests ; 3 of the 15-year tests correct ; fails the first and third, which are memory tests. (It should be noted that extremely good records were made on most of the Binet tests ; the answers were very quick and relevant.) **Construction Test I :** 13" ; 8 moves. **Construction Test II :** 1' 1" ; 16 moves. **Tapping Test :** 52 and 60 squares, first and second trial respectively, no errors. **Pictorial Completion Test :** 2' 50" ; 3 logical errors. **Cross Line Test I :** Correct first trial. **Cross Line Test II :** Correct first trial. **Arbitrary Association Test :** No errors. **Easy Opposites Test :** No errors or failures ; average time 1.3". **Visual Memory Span** — reproduction of Binet figures : Drawn correctly. **Visual Memory Span** — for numerals : 6 numerals correct. **Auditory Memory Span for numerals :** 4 numerals correct in each of the three trials, 5 numerals correct twice in six trials ; 6 numerals a failure. **Auditory Memory Span for Syllables :** 16 syllables correct, 18 syllables failure. **Memory for Logical Material** — visual verbal presentation : 13 out of 20 items, correct sequence, fair verbal accuracy. **Memory for Logical Material** — auditory verbal presentation : 11 items out of 12, sequence correct, fair verbal accuracy. (Says, "I saw this like a picture when it was read to me.") **Aussage Test :** Very full and accurate free account, showing good powers of perception ; good account in response to questions ; accepts 2 out of 7 suggestions offered. **Analogies Test :** 4 of 5 problems correct. **Terman Arithmetical Reasoning Test :** All 3 problems correct. **Continuous Subtraction Test :** 7 from 100, 1' 7" ; no errors. (Toward the end made one mistake, later said "I made one mistake ; it should have been ", etc. and corrected it.) **Test for Auditory Perception :** Fails to repeat correctly difficult sentences. (See case-study,

p. 95, for details.) **School Work** : Arithmetic : Adds four 3-place numerals correctly. Knows the combinations of the multiplication table ; subtracts correctly ; cannot do long division. (It should be remembered that because of special defect in reading he never went farther than the 4th grade.) See, also, Terman Arithmetical Reasoning and Continuous Subtraction Test. Writing : Writes a good, legible hand. Spelling : Writes from dictation " Dog run on steerts " ; " The gril go to school " ; " The print mad soom card." (Was uncertain whether " print " was " painter " or " printer.") Reading : On 2nd-grade passage fails on many words, such as " heart ", " leaves ", " often ", " twig ", etc. On 3rd-grade passage shows much hesitancy, fails on many words. 5th-grade passage practically a failure. Makes some effort to read with expression ; reproduction quite good.

Case 15. JAMES M. 15 years, 2 months.
Introductory Test : 1'. **Construction Test I** : 1' 7", 29 moves. **Puzzle Box** : 2' 10" ; 1 error ; good result, logical procedure. **Tapping Test** : 88 and 89 squares first and second trials respectively; 1 and 4 errors. **Cross Line Test I** : Correct on first trial. **Cross Line Test II** : Correct on second trial. **Code Test** : 4 errors ; 3 dots omitted. **Easy Opposites Test** : 3 errors ; average time 1.1". **Visual Memory Span — reproduction of Binet figures** : Both incorrect first trial ; correct second trial. (For details see case-study, p. 98.) **Memory for Logical Material — visual verbal presentation** : 16 items out of 20, incorrect sequence. (For details see case-study.) **Memory for Logical Material — auditory presentation** : 10 items out of 12 correct ; only 1 item not in logical sequence. **School Work** : Adds, subtracts, multiplies, and divides correctly. Writes from dictation " The printer made some cards." Reading : 5th-grade passage read very poorly, fails on many words, including such simple ones as " field ", " shore, " " crib", etc.

Case 16. WALTER Z. 11 years old.
Introductory Test : 1' 19". **Construction Test I** : Failure ; very poor attempt. **Construction Test II** : 44", 11

moves ; very good record. **Puzzle Box** : 2′ 3″, 3 errors. **Instructions Box** : Correct on second trial. **Cross Line Test I** : Failure on third trial. **Cross Line Test II** : Failure on third trial. **Visual Memory — reproduction of Binet figures:** Extremely well done. **Arbitrary Association Test** : No errors. **School Work** : Cannot read ; does not know letters. Arithmetic : Adds two single digits, *e.g.* 4 + 2 = 6.

Second Testing 1 year later :

Binet grade : Through 9 years. Failures : 8 years, (2) and (4) ; 9 years, (2) and (4) ; 10 years, (3) and (5) ; 12 years, (2), (3), (4), (5). **Cross Line Test I** : Correct first trial. **Cross Line Test II** : Correct first trial. **School Work** : Reading : Recognized only two words in 1st-grade passage. Writes from dictation " I see the cat ", but no more difficult sentence.

Third Testing 2 years after last testing :

Binet grade : All of 10-year and 3 of 12-year tests correct. Failures : 12-years, (4) and (5). **Construction Test I** : 1′ 45″, 28 moves. (Of these only one move was an impossibility.) **Construction Test II** : 23″, 11 moves. **Puzzle Box:** 36″, very well done. **Cross Line Test I** : Correct first trial. **Code Test** : Failure (6 errors). **Pictorial Completion Test:** 3′ 28″, 1 logical error. **Arbitrary Association Test** : No errors. **Auditory Memory Span** : 6 numerals correct. **Memory for Logical Material — auditory verbal presentation** : 9 of 12 items, good logical sequence, but poorly expressed. **School Work** : Reading : Fails on nearly all words of 1st-grade passage. Writing and Spelling : In writing from dictation " The boy went to school ", does not attempt the words " went " and " school." Writes a firm, legible hand. Arithmetic : Adds column of five 1-place numerals correctly ; does not know process of carrying.

Fourth Testing 2 years after last testing :

Binet grade : All 12-year tests correct ; all 15-year tests correct except (3). **Easy Opposites Test** : 3 errors, average time 2.1″. **School Work** : Reading : In simple passage fails on such words as " fast ", " were ", " cold ", etc. Reads 1st-grade passage haltingly ; fails on " dig ", " elephant."

Says he cannot read the newspaper, " there are too many long words." Writing and Spelling : Writes from dictation " The girl went to school " ; " The beard make som cars" (The printer made some cards). He has learned to write correctly a number of difficult words, *e.g.*, " Washington ", " Mississippi ", and " Constantinople." Says he has consciously learned to remember how these words " look." Arithmetic : Adds correctly. Adds money, makes change, does orally simple problems involving money. Has never been taught multiplication and division.

Case 17. HAROLD N. 11 years old.
Binet grade : Passes all of the 10-year and 2 of the 12-year tests. Fails 12 year, (3) and (4), (5) not given. (Notably good answers to common-sense questions, quick detection of absurdities, good language ability.) **Introductory Test** : 2' 2''. **Construction Test I** : 2' 57'' ; 22 moves. (One hour later does this in 12'', 5 moves.) **Construction Test II** : 2' 49'' ; 22 moves. (Thoughtfully done ; rational trial and error method ; no repetition of errors.) **Cross Line Test I** : Correct on second trial. **Cross Line Test II** : Correct on second trial. **Pictorial Completion Test** : 4' 2'' ; 1 logical and 1 illogical error. **Arbitrary Association Test** : No errors. **Aussage** : gives good functional account ; on cross-examination, many details. **Visual Memory — reproduction of Binet figures** : Correct. **Auditory Memory Span** : 6 numerals correct. **Memory for Logical Material — auditory verbal presentation** : 7 out of 12 items. Incorrect logical sequence. (Used as test for remote memory 48 hours later, 6 out of 12 items.) **Memory for Logical Material — visual verbal presentation** : Not given, cannot read passage.

Tests for remote memory 5 days after first trial: **Construction Test I** : 28'', 10 moves. Fails to place correctly numerals on figure **Cross Line Test I**. Draws correctly 1 out of 2 Binet geometrical figures ; cannot remember the other figure. Sings correctly melody and words of song learned in school. Remembers correctly 6 of the 9 simple geometric forms of the arbitrary association test.

School Work : Arithmetic : Adds correctly single column figures ; knows simple number combinations ; gives correct answer to simple problems, *e.g.* : If 3 cost 15 cents, how much would 2 cost? If 9 apples were divided equally among 3 children, how many would each receive? Adds correctly a quarter, a dime, a nickel, and a penny, etc. Spelling : Writes his own name correctly. Cannot write any sentence from dictation. Writes " run ", " nam " (man), " can ", " onj " (and). Says his teacher has made him write these many times. One week later misspells his surname in writing it ; orally spells it correctly. Cannot identify all the letters of the alphabet. Reading : Fails to read first grade passage; knows only " I can." Reads numerals.

Second Testing 9 months later:

School Work : Has learned the multiplication tables. Still cannot write any sentence from dictation or any from his own invention. Has learned to write four words, namely, " man ", " can ", " his ", " and." Reading : Fails on 1st-grade passage. Doesn't know the following words : " Not ", " am ", " dig." Remote Memory : Retells details of picture used in Aussage test fully and well.

Third Testing 1 month later:

Writes " ral " for " rat ", " see " for " the." Reading : No improvement. General information quite fair for opportunities. Conversational ability normal. Record in manual training room very good ; is said by teacher to copy well, to follow directions, and to have quite a little ability to plan and invent.

Case 18. RICHARD T. 15 years.

Binet grade : All 10-year and three 12-year tests correct. Failure : 12 years, (4) ; (5) not given. Construction Test I: 12″, 6 moves. Construction Test II : 13″, 11 moves. Cross Line Test I : Correct first trial. Cross Line Test II : Correct first trial. Pictorial Completion Test : 3′ 37″ ; 2 logical and 1 illogical error. Visual Memory — reproduction of Binet figures : Correctly drawn. Aussage Test : Gives very full but quite inaccurate recital. Suggestible. School Work:

Reading : 3rd-grade passage read poorly ; fails on all but simplest words. Writing and Spelling : Writes from dictation " The boy went to school." Arithmetic : Adds four 3-place numerals correctly. Subtracts and multiplies correctly.

Case 19. THOMAS S. 15 years.
Introductory Test : 3' 5" ; much of time spent on triangles. Construction Test I : 3', 26 moves. Cross Line Test I : Correct first trial. Cross Line Test II : Correct third trial. School Work : Writes from dictation " The pre made soom c." (The printer made some cards). Arithmetic : Adds 3-place numerals and multiplies promptly.
Second Testing one day later :
Construction Test II : 40", 11 moves. Puzzle Box : 1' 45", 1 error. Tapping Test : 70 and 77 squares respectively at first and second trial ; no errors. Arbitrary Association Test : No errors. Memory for Logical Material — auditory verbal presentation : 11 of 12 items given ; incorrect logical sequence. Peculiarly disconnected, short phrases ; English very poor. Easy Opposites : 3 failures ; average time 2.7". School Work : Reads some few monosyllables only.
Third Testing three months later :
Reading : Somewhat better ; knows a few more words, but fails on three words (elephant, dig, ground) in four lines of a 1st-grade passage. Writing and spelling : Writes from dictation " See the dog on the Street ", "The cat rouns fast."

Case 20. RUPERT N. 16 years.
Construction Test I : 20", 5 moves. Construction Test II : 1' 4", 12 moves. Cross Line Test I : Correct first trial. Cross Line Test II : Correct first trial. Pictorial Completion Test : 2', 1 logical error. School Work : Reading : Reads 3rd-grade passage fairly well ; all words read correctly ; not much expression ; reproduction fairly good. Writing and Spelling : Writes from dictation " The pter made son cards " (The printer made some cards), " I neear waet ene plaes atsed in Chicago " (I never went any place outside of Chicago).

Arithmetic : Adds correctly ; in long division makes one careless error ; multiplies simple numbers ; fails on tables of 7's and 8's.

Second Testing five days later :

Binet grade : Through 10 years. Failures : 10 years, (5) ; 12 years, (1), (2), (4), (5). **Puzzle Box :** 1′ 9″, 2 errors. **Tapping Test :** 74 and 73 squares respectively, first and second trial, 0 and 2 errors respectively. **Cross Line Test II :** Correct first trial. (Lettering changed from arrangement used previously.) **Visual Memory — reproduction of Binet figures :** Correct. **Easy Opposites :** 6 errors, 2 failures ; average time 2.8″; range 1.4″–7.8″.

Third Testing one week after second testing :

Code Test : 3 errors on first trial (was not trying) ; 1 error on second trial.

Fourth Testing four months after third testing :

Binet : All the 10-year tests correct. Failures : 12 years, (4) and (5) ; 15 years, (1), (2), (4). **Easy Opposites** (new list of words) : 1 error ; average time 1.9″ ; range 1″–5.″ **Kraepelin Subtraction Test :** Subtracting 7 from 100 ; 3′ 42″, 1 error. Subtracting 4 from 51, 2′, 1 error. **School Work :** Writes from dictation " The priter mead sen cerds " (The printer made some cards). Arithmetic : Adds and subtracts correctly.

Case 21. HENRY J. 16 years.

Binet : All 10-year tests correct. 12-year tests, failed only on (4). **Construction Test II :** 36″, 11 moves. **Cross Line Test I :** Correct on first trial. **Cross Line Test II :** Correct on second trial. **Code Test :** 4 errors. **Easy Opposites :** 1 error, average time 1.6.″ **Arbitrary Association Test :** No errors. **Memory for Logical Material — visual verbal presentation :** 15 of 20 items given in logical sequence. **Memory for Logical Material — auditory verbal presentation :** 11 of 12 items given, slight changes in logical sequence. (Retells correctly stories told in Binet absurdities test.) **Auditory Memory Span :** 4 numerals only. Fails on 5 numerals in each of six trials. **Visual Memory Span : 5**

numerals correct. Cannot remember two telephone numbers of 4 numerals each. **Memory Span for Syllables :** 14 syllables correct. One slight error on both 16 and 18 syllables. **School Work :** Reads 3rd-grade passage fairly well ; gives good reproduction. Writes from dictation " The boy goes to school ", " The printer made some cards." Adds, subtracts, multiplies, and divides correctly.

Case 22. BENJAMIN L. 20 years old.

Binet : Through 12 and 15-year tests correctly. All adult tests correct except (5). Tests involving mental representation, *i.e.* adult (1) and (2), correct only slowly and with difficulty. **Construction Test I :** 11″, 5 moves. **Construction Test II :** 33″, 11 moves. **Cross Line Test I :** Correct first trial. **Cross Line Test II :** Correct first trial. **Code Test :** 2 errors. **Pictorial Completion Test :** 2′ 50″, 2 illogical errors. (It should be added that this test presents certain definite features for adults. For discussion see Psych. Rev., May, 1914.) **Opposites Test :** No errors or failures, average time 1″. **Association Test, object — attribute :** No errors or failures ; average time 1.5″. **Memory for Logical Material — visual verbal presentation :** 19 of 20 items given, correct logical sequence, only slight verbal changes. (Compare with failure on adult (5) Binet.) **Memory for Logical Material — auditory verbal presentation :** 11 of 12 items given, correct logical sequence, only slight verbal changes. **Visual Memory Span :** 9 numerals correct. Reproduction of Binet figures : correct. **Auditory Memory Span :** 12 numerals correct ; 13 numerals, one numeral transposed. **Memory Span for Syllables :** 32 syllables correct. (Not tried further.) **Hard Directions Test :** 3′ 5″, no errors. **Analogies Test :** Four correct ; 1 error. **Terman Arithmetical Reasoning Test :** 1 correct ; 2 failures. **Terman Ball and Field Test :** Correct. **Terman Link Chain Test :** Correct.

Case 23. PETER R. 11 years old.

Introductory Test : 56″. **Construction Test I :** 46″, 16 moves. **Construction Test II :** 1′ 1″, 21 moves. **Pictorial**

Completion Test : 4′ 27″, 1 logical and 1 illogical error.
Cross Line Test II : Correct first trial. **Arbitrary Association Test** : 3 errors. **Memory for Logical Material** — auditory verbal presentation : 10 of 12 items given, logical sequence and verbal accuracy good. **School Work** : Reading :
only a few words of 1st-grade passage read. Writing and
Spelling : Writes own name poorly and three words, " The
cat run." Arithmetic : Adds single column of four numerals
by counting on fingers ; cannot subtract ; gives the tables
of 2's and 3's by adding on fingers and by making marks.
Asked how much is $1.00 less 60 cents, makes one hundred
marks, counts off sixty and then counts the remainder.

Second Testing following day :

Binet grade : 9¾ years. Failures : 8-year, (4) ; 9-year,
(4) ; 10-year, (3) and (4) ; 12-year, (3), (4) and (5). **Memory
Span for Numerals** : 6 correct. **Construction Test I** : 13″ ;
5 moves. **Cross Line Test I** : Correct on first trial,
(promptly). **Arbitrary Association Test** : No errors.

Third Testing 10 months later :

Binet grade : 9⅖. Failures : the same as previously,
except 10-year (3) now correct, 12-year (2) now failure.
Cross Line Test II : Correct on first trial. **Pictorial Completion Test** : 2′ 53″, 1 logical error. **Arbitrary Association
Test** : Correct. (All these tests given to find whether any
deterioration or improvement.) **Easy Opposites Test** : 2
errors, average time 1.8″. **School Work** : Reading : No
improvement, reads only very few of even simple words.
Writing and Spelling : Has added no new words to writing
vocabulary. Arithmetic : Still adds a column of single
figures by counting ; no new process learned. **General Information** : Exceedingly poor ; knows the president in office,
but not who preceded him nor who was first president ;
cannot tell time ; cannot tell year in which born, although
knows present year and own age ; cannot name the month,
nor the day of the week ; knows nothing about the city,
except how to reach the laboratory from his home ; geographical and historical items all failures.

Fourth Testing 3 months later :

Binet grade : same as previously. **Terman Scale** : Passes 9-year tests and 10-year (4). **Visual Memory** — reproduction of Binet and other figures : correct. **Cross Line Test II** (renumbered) : Correct on first trial. **Instructions Box** : Failure on third trial due to inability to find the numbers on the dial ; other steps of process correct. **Auditory Memory for Syllables** : 20 correct. **School Work** : No improvement in reading or spelling. Arithmetic : Has improved in addition ; has learned the process of carrying, but fails in subtraction ; has learned the simpler combinations of multiplication table, but fails on difficult ones. Makes simple change, *e.g.*, 50 ¢ less 27 ¢, correct, but fails on $1.00 less 66 ¢.

Fifth Testing 1 month later :

Re-testing on failures in the Binet series, still fails 8-year (4), but now gives 9-year (4) correctly ; gives correctly 12-year (2) ; still fails 12-year (3) and (4), but makes better record than ever before on (3). **Memory Span for Numerals** : 6 numerals correct, one trial in three ; 7 numerals complete failure. **Memory for Syllables** : 24 correct, fails on 26. **Knox Cube Test** : Parts (a) (b) (c) correct on first trial ; part (d) correct on second trial ; part (e) correct on third trial. **Special Tests for Remote Memory** (besides the various tests given above) : Fails completely to remember the simple geometric figures of the substitution test, which he has had three separate times. Fails to remember any of the passages used for testing immediate auditory verbal memory, — does not even remember that he had such a test a year previously. Fails to tell time, birthday, the current month, etc., in spite of recent intensive training. Remembers vaguely parts of Construction Test II, but relationships extremely poor. For other items see the text. **Aussage** : Gives good free account enumerating all the prominent objects and some of the less prominent ones ; on cross-examination gives many more details. Somewhat inaccurate, adds fictional items, not suggestible. **Recognition Memory** : Shown 5 pictures, selects them promptly from among ten later presented. **General Information** : Still fails to tell time ; fails to give the date ; cannot tell his birthday. **School Work** : Fails on simple problem in multiplication ; does simple example in subtraction in which he has had drill just two days previously ; solves correctly problem, " If you make $4.00 a week and spend $2.00 a week, how long would it take you to save $6.00? "

Case 24. HARRY R. 14 years, 9 months.

Binet grade : Through 12 years. Failures : 9-year, (4) ; 10-year, (2) ; passes 15-year (1), (4), and (5). Construction Test I : Failure in 5'. Construction Test II : Failure in 5'. Cross Line Test I : Failure on 4th trial. Cross Line Test II : Failure on 4th trial. Pictorial Completion Test : 3' 20", 1 logical error. Easy Opposites Test : No errors or failure ; average time 2.2." Arbitrary Association Test : 3 errors. Auditory Memory Span : 8 numerals correct. Visual Memory Span — reproduction of Binet figures : Failure. Reproduction of two other figures similar in character, failure ; cannot draw façade of own house ; cannot draw floor plan of own home. Memory for Syllables : Reproduced 24 syllables correctly. Memory for Logical Material — visual verbal presentation : 12 of 20 items, correct sequence, fair verbal accuracy. Memory for Logical Material — auditory verbal presentation : 10 of 12 items, good verbal accuracy. School Work : Arithmetic : (Oral.) Knows combinations in addition and multiplication ; makes 1 error in adding four 3-place numerals. Subtraction correct ; long division, process correct, but several inaccuracies. Problems ; at 36 ¢ a dozen 4 cost 12 ¢, etc., promptly. Writing : Writes a fair, legible hand ; writes from dictation " The prenter mad some cors." Reading : 3rd grade passage read slowly ; numerous inaccuracies ; fails on fairly simple words, e.g., " frightened " ; called saw " snow ", etc. Reproduction good. Catch phrases correctly repeated.

Case 25. EDGAR M. 11 years.

Binet : All tests through 15-year age-level correct except 12-year (4). 12-year (3), correct only on second trial. Construction Test I : 1' 25", 14 moves. Construction Test II : 1' 3", 13 moves. Puzzle Box : 4' 1", 2 errors. (1' 55" spent in studying situation.) 5' 20" to put box together again. **Tapping Test** : 48 and 56 squares, respectively, first and second trial, no errors. **Cross Line Test I** : Correct on first trial. **Cross Line Test II** : Correct on first trial. **Pictorial Completion Test** : 5' 4", no errors. (Much time required to find the correct pieces. Perceptions slow ; apperceptions rapid.) **Arbitrary Association Test** : No errors ; 1' 57" required to place numerals in learning part. **Visual Memory Span** : 6 numerals correct with one exposure ; 7 numerals correct with two exposures ; 8 numerals correct with three exposures. (Translates probably into auditory terms.) **Auditory Memory Span** : 8 numerals correct, one reading. **Memory for Logical Material — visual verbal presentation** : 13 of 20 items given ; correct logical sequence. **Memory for Logical Material — auditory verbal presentation** : 11 of 12 items given ; correct logical sequence. **Easy Opposites Test** : No errors or failures ; average time 1.4". **Easy Directions Test** : 4' 32", 1 error. **Hard Directions Test** : Time ? no errors. **Analogies Test** : All correct. **Aussage** : Free recital, 5 items. Cross-examination, 14 items correct ; 7 errors ; replies " Don't know " 9 times, and " Not sure " 2 times. Denies seeing two prominent objects ; no suggestions accepted. **School Work** : Reading : 5th-grade passage fluent, but tires of it. Spelling and Writing : Spelling comparatively poor. Writes very slowly and poorly ; requires much effort. (Spelling taught him by writing ; oral recitations only once a week.) Arithmetic : Adds, subtracts, multiplies correctly. Fails on long division. Makes change slowly. Fails on simple problems, *e.g.*, At 48 cents a dozen, how much would 5 cost? Enjoys French lessons ; does well ; this subject taught entirely by auditory method. Fond of music, good sense of rhythm.

Case 26. MELVIN W. 15 years.

Binet grade : Through 12-year tests ; no failures. **Construction Test I** : Failure in 5'. **Construction Test II** : 4' 6", 40 moves ; trial and error method ; many repetitions of errors. **Puzzle Box** : Failure in 10' ; correct, after many

errors, in 11′ 1″. **Cross Line Test I** : Correct on first trial.
Cross Line Test II : Correct on first trial. **Pictorial Completion Test** : 3′ 5″ ; 1 logical and 1 illogical error. **Auditory Memory Span** : 6 numerals correct. **Visual Memory —** reproduction of Binet figures : Correctly done. **School Work** : Reading, 3rd-grade passage read poorly ; fails on longer words. Writing and Spelling : Writes from dictation " The preuter maid som cards " (The printer made some cards). Arithmetic : One error in adding four 3-place numerals. Short division correct. Errors in subtraction. Fails on long division. Knows multiplication tables.

Second Testing three months later :
Introductory Test : 1′ 10″. **Construction Test I** : 14″, 6 moves. (Probably due to accident.) **Construction Test II** : Failure in 5′. **Puzzle Box** : 1′ 9″ ; 2 errors ; cannot put the box together. **Stenquist Tests** : All models copied in 27′. **Terman Ball and Field Test** : Very poor failure. **Yerkes Multiple Choice Test** : Problem I, correct on 18th trial. Problem II, correct on 15th trial. Problem III, correct on 10th trial. Problem IV, correct on 5th trial. **Tapping Test** : 59 and 56 squares respectively, first and second trial ; 8 errors on first trial, 0 errors on second. (Made very great effort.) **Arbitrary Association Test** : No errors. **Memory for Logical Material** — auditory verbal presentation : 10 of 12 items given ; correct logical sequence ; English poor. **Easy Opposites Test** : 1 error ; average time 1.6″. **Woodworth-Wells Easy Directions Test** : 1′ 58″, 3 errors. **Terman Arithmetical Reasoning Test** : Correct (2 out of 3). **School Work** : Reading, some improvement on 3rd-grade passage ; fewer words mispronounced, but read haltingly. Writing and Spelling : Writes from dictation " The printer made some cards." Arithmetic : Adds and subtracts correctly examples previously failed. Multiplies correctly. Has not yet learned long division.

Case 27. ALEXANDER T. 13 years, 9 months.
Binet grade : Correct through 12 years, except 12, (4).
Construction Test I : 4′ 30″, 56 moves (of these 14 were

impossibilities). **Construction Test II** : Failure in 5'. **Stenquist Test** : Failure in 30' ; errors on the lock, and the star was a failure. **Tapping Test** : 76 and 69 squares 1st and 2nd trials respectively, and 0 and 1 error respectively. **Instructions Box** : Correct on second trial. **Cross Line Test I**: Correct 1st trial. **Cross Line Test II** : Correct 1st trial. **Pictorial Completion Test** : 2' 15", 2 logical errors. **School Work** : Arithmetic : Does long division correctly. Writing : Writes rapid legible hand. Spelling : Writes " The printer made some cards." Reading : 5th-grade passage read fluently.

Case 28. ARTHUR R. 17 years.

(Testing done on two days, one immediately following the other, reported together.)

Binet : 12-year tests all correct, but (2) very slowly answered ; (3), 60 words in 2' 30". 15-year tests : fails on (1) and (3) ; (5) answered very slowly. Adult tests : (2) solved when allowed to ponder overnight ; (3) slowly and poorly done ; (4) slowly and poorly done.

Construction Test I : 1' 18", 12 moves. **Construction Test II** : 2' 2", 26 moves. **Puzzle Box** : 6' 12". (5' study before first move made ; then only 1 error, though 1' 12" required to complete.) **Tapping Test** : 98 and 101 squares respectively, first and second trials, 0 and 5 errors respectively. **Pictorial Completion Test** : 3' 35". No errors. (Very slow reactions for age.) **Arbitrary Association Test**: 2 errors on first trial ; no errors on second trial. **Visual Memory** — reproduction of Binet figures : Correct. **Auditory Memory Span** : 6 numerals correct. **Memory for Logical Material** — visual verbal presentation : 16 of 20 items given ; correct sequence. **Memory for Logical Material** — auditory verbal presentation : 10 of 12 items given, 2 items transposed. **Easy Opposites Test** : No errors or failures, average time 1.6". **Kraepelin Subtraction Test** : Subtracting 7 from 100 ; 1' 13", no errors. **Terman Link Chain Test** : Failure first day ; solved correctly overnight. **Terman Ball and Field Test** : Poor attempt. **Sharp's Ethical**

Questions answered very slowly, but fully comprehended.
School Work : Reading : excellent. Writing and Spelling :
Writes from dictation " The printer made some cards."
Arithmetic : Adds nine 3-place numerals correctly, but
slowly ; long division, 1 error.

Case 29. AGNES Z. 8 years.
Binet grade : Through 7 years. Failures : 5 years, (1) ;
6 years, (3) ; 7 years, (4) ; 8 years, (1), (2), (4) ; 9 years,
all except (2). Drawing of square showed poor coördinations ; attempts at drawing rhomboid very poor. **Introductory Test** : Failure ; correct in 2' except for triangles.
Shown how to place pieces of triangle, fails after four trials.
Construction Test I : 15", 7 moves. Result evidently accidental. Immediate retrial failure. **Arbitrary Association
Test** : Makes many errors in placing figures with model
before her. **Pictorial Completion Test** : (Not given with
standard procedure.) Gives meaning of situations very well
for age. **Auditory Memory Span** : 5 numerals correct.
Memory Span for Syllables : 16 syllables correct. Recites
Stevenson's " The Shadow " correctly ; cannot give meaning. **School Work** : Reading, 1st and 2nd grade passages
read well. Writing and Spelling : Writing almost illegible ;
spells simple words orally without errors. Arithmetic : Adds
combinations of two numbers up to 12, *e.g.*, 7 + 3, 6 + 6,
etc.

Case 30. LEONARD B. 17 years, 11 months.
Introductory Test : 1' 54", of which 54" was spent on
triangles. **Construction Test I** : 33", 7 moves. **Construction Test II** : 55", 14 moves. **Cross Line Test I** : Correct
on second trial. **Cross Line Test II** : Failure after four
trials ; cannot draw from memory figure used.
Second Testing two days later:
Binet : All 12-year tests correct except (5) ; 15 years,
failure (2) and (3) ; adult tests, all failures. **Puzzle Box** :
4' 4", 3 errors. **Tapping Test** : 87 and 90 squares respectively on first and second trial, 0 and 1 error, respectively.

Pictorial Completion Test : 5′ 54″ ; 1 logical and 1 illogical error. **Easy Opposites Test :** 1 failure ; average time 1.8″. **Kraepelin Subtraction Test :** Subtracting 7 from 100, 2′, 6 errors. **Arbitrary Association Test :** 2 errors. (Both figures left unnumbered ; 1 and 9 evidently confused.) **Cross Line Test I :** Failure after two trials. **Visual Memory — reproduction of Binet figures :** Failure after eight trials each after new exposure. (Copies figures correctly ; cannot even after this draw them from memory.) **Memory for Logical Material — visual verbal presentation :** 14 of 20 items given ; correct sequence. **Memory for Logical Material — auditory verbal presentation :** 8 of 12 items given ; correct sequence. **Instructions Box :** Correct only on fifth trial. **Terman Ball and Field Test :** Very well done. **Cancellation Test :** Well done ; rapid, accurate reactions. **Aussage :** Free recital, 11 items ; cross examination, 12 items correct ; 5 errors ; answers " Don't know " on 4 items. **School Work :** 6th-grade passage read fluently. **Writing and Spelling :** Writes from dictation " The printer made some cards ", but " The revoluntary war was carried on largely under the auspieces of the Continaltal Congress." **Arithmetic :** Adds five 4-place numerals correctly : fails on long division ; fails to add fractions. Oral problems : fails on such examples as $8 + 7 + 5 - 2 \times 2$, and other similar ones. Asked if 1 dozen apples cost 54 cents, how much will 8 apples cost, gives steps required, but cannot solve.

Third Testing one week later :

Puzzle Box : 2′, 3 errors. Rapidly put box together again. **Cannot draw recognizable representation** of simple ink-bottle.

Case 31. JULIAN M. 14 years.

Binet : (1908 series used). All 10, 11, and 12-year tests correct. **Introductory Test :** 1′ 20″. **Construction Test I :** Failure ; 60 moves. **Construction Test II :** 1′ 10″ (result possibly accidental). **Puzzle Box :** 7′, many errors, first correct move made at 6′. **Instructions Box :** Correct on third trial. **Tapping Test :** 82 and 83 squares, respectively, on first and second trial ; 20 and 5 errors respectively. **Cross Line Test I** : Correct on first trial. **Cross Line Test II** : Correct on first trial. **Code Test** : Failure. 3 symbols wrong and 6 dots omitted. **Pictorial Completion Test** : Time? 3 logical and 4 illogical errors. Apperceptions very defective. **Arbitrary Association Test** : No errors. **Checkers**, fails to take advantage of obvious chances. **School Work** : Reading : 6th-grade passage read fluently, with good expression. Writing and Spelling : Writes from dictation "The printer made some cards." Arithmetic : Adds seven 4-place numbers correctly, but slowly. Fails on long division ; makes errors in subtraction ; says $18 - 6 = 3$. Asked if $2\frac{1}{2}$ pounds cost 45 cents, how much will $3\frac{1}{2}$ cost? answers $6.08. Poorly informed in regard to historical, geographical, and local facts.

Case 32. ALICE J. 13 years, 6 months.
Introductory Test : 31″. **Construction Test I** : 36″, 17 moves. **Construction Test II** : 6′ 43″, 58 moves. (Scored as failure.) **Cross Line Test I** : Correct on first trial. **Cross Line Test II** : Correct on first trial. **Pictorial Completion Test** : 2′ 18″ ; 2 logical errors. **Arbitrary Association Test** : No errors. **Tapping Test** : 44 squares in each of two trials ; 1 and 0 errors respectively. **School Work** : Reading : 5th-grade passage read well ; occasionally slight hesitation. Writing and Spelling : Writes from dictation " The printer made some cards." Arithmetic : Adds, subtracts, multiplies, divides correctly ; adds fractions.

Second Testing three weeks later :
Construction Test II : 33″, 13 moves. **Tapping Test** : 63 and 70 squares respectively ; 8 and 7 errors respectively. (Was urged to do better than previously. Made great effort.)

Case 33. MORGAN G. 14 years.
Binet grade : Through 12-year tests without any failures. **Introductory Test** : 1′ 7″ ; 22″ spent on triangles. **Construction Test I** : Failure in 5′. (1 hour later 1′ 54″, 15 moves.) **Construction Test II** : 56″, 14 moves. **Cross Line**

Test I : Correct on first trial. **Cross Line Test II** : Correct on first trial. **Pictorial Completion Test** : 2′ 54″, no errors. **Easy Opposites Test** : 2 errors ; average time 2.3 ″ ; range 1.2″ to 7.8″. **Kraepelin Subtraction Test** : Subtracting 7 from 100, all wrong ; 4 from 41, 1′ 10″, 4 errors. (Toward the end counts by ones.) 3 from 51, 57″, 5 errors. (Failed again on this test one month later. Then subtracting 7 from 101, all failure ; continuous addition by 7, beginning with 2, 2′ 20″, 3 errors.) **Tapping Test** : 60 and 57 squares respectively on first and second trial ; 3 and 5 errors respectively. **School Work** : Reading : 3rd-grade passage fairly well read ; knows all words ; somewhat jerky in manner ; reproduction correct. Writing and Spelling : Writes from dictation " The boy goes to school." Arithmetic : Long division correct.

Case 34. HENRY B. 17 years.
Binet : All 10 and 12-year tests done promptly ; on 15-year tests fails on (3) and (5). **Construction Test I** : 27″, 9 moves. **Construction Test II** : 1′ 57″, 17 moves. **Cross Line Test II** : Correct on first trial. **Pictorial Completion Test** : 3′ 12″ ; 2 logical errors. **Tapping Test** : 62 and 80 squares respectively on first and second trial ; 3 and 4 errors respectively. **Easy Opposites Test** : 2 errors and 2 failures ; average time 2.3″ ; range 1.2″ to 6.6″. Second trial (new list of words) ; 1 error and 2 failures ; average time 2.7″ ; range 1.2″ to 9.8″. **Kraepelin Subtraction Test** : Subtracting 7 from 100, 1′ 53″, 2 errors. (Frequently says, " I get mixed up ", or " What did I say last ? ") Subtracting 6 from 75, 1′ 31″, 3 errors. **Memory for Logical Material — visual verbal presentation** : 14 of 20 items given ; logical sequence, but with little verbal accuracy. **Memory for Logical Material — auditory verbal presentation** : 8 of 12 items given ; incorrect sequence and little verbal accuracy. **Woodworth-Wells Easy Directions Test** : 2′ 55″, 2 errors ; 3′ 54″, 2 errors, second set. **Woodworth-Wells Hard Directions Test** : 5′ 13″, 8 errors. (Could not keep mind on work ; said he was not fatigued.) **Analogies Test** : 4 correct, 1 wrong. **Terman Arithmetical Reasoning Test** : All three correct.

School Work : Writing and Spelling : Writes from dictation " I hereby apply for a position." Arithmetic : Does long division correctly ; cannot do problem in interest.

Case 35. CELIA K. 17 years.

Binet grade : All 12-year tests correct except (5) ; that not given because cannot read English. **Construction Test I** : 12″, 7 moves. **Cross Line Test I** : Correct on first trial. **Cross Line Test II** : Correct on first trial. **Pictorial Completion Test** : 3′ 56″ ; 1 logical and 1 illogical error. **Tapping Test** : 72 and 79 squares respectively on first and second trial, 3 and 2 errors respectively. **School Work** : Reads little English ; has never attended English speaking school. Writing and Spelling : Writes from dictation " The cat run." Arithmetic : Adds, subtracts, multiplies correctly ; makes careless errors in division.

Second Testing four months later :

Construction Test II : 1′ 30″, 18 moves. **School Work** : ׳ Reading : Fails on many words in 1st-grade passage. Writing and Spelling : Writes from dictation " The boy goes to school." Arithmetic : Does problem in long division correctly. Fails to make change.

Third Testing two months after last testing :

Tapping Test : 73 and 76 squares respectively on first and second trial, 3 and 0 errors respectively. **Easy Opposites Test** : No error or failure ; average time 1.8″. **Kraepelin Subtraction Test** : Subtracting 6 from 75 ; 52″, 1 error. **Cross Line Test II** : Correct on first trial. **Counts backward 20 to 0** in 14″ ; counts months backward 20″.

Case 36. JULIA D. 15 years.

Introductory Test : 2′ 10″. **Construction Test I** : 5″, 5 moves. **Construction Test II** : 1′ 40″, 25 moves. **Cross Line Test I**: Correct on first׳ trial. **Cross Line Test II** : Correct on second trial. **Code Test** : Failure. **Pictorial Completion Test** : 2′ 58″ ; 2 logical errors. **Arbitrary Association Test** : No errors.

Second Testing nineteen months later :

Cross Line Test II : Correct on first trial. **Pictorial Completion Test** : 1′ 30″, no errors. **Opposites Test** : No errors or failure ; average time 2.2″. **Kraepelin Subtraction Test:** Subtracting 7 from 100 ; 1′ 4″, no errors.

Case 37. OLIVER L. 17 years.
Construction Test I : 35″, 9 moves. **Construction Test II** : 47″, 13 moves. **Cross Line Test II** : Correct on first trial. **Code Test** : No symbols wrong, 6 dots omitted ; done rapidly ; good method used. **Pictorial Completion Test:** 2′ 19″, 2 logical errors. **Tapping Test** : 85 and 87 squares respectively on first and second trial ; 1 and 0 errors respectively. **Easy Opposites Test** : No errors or failure ; average time 1.3″. **Memory for Logical Material — visual verbal presentation :** 17 of 20 items given ; correct sequence. **Memory for Logical Material — auditory verbal presentation :** 11 of 12 items given ; correct sequence.

Case 38. ALLEN B. 13 years.
Binet : All 10 and 12-year tests correct except 12-year (2). (Becomes almost hysterical at absurdities test ; laughs uncontrolledly.) **Construction Test I** : 1′ 27″, 20 moves. **Construction Test II** : Failure on first trial ; failure on second trial, short time after first. **Cross Line Test I :** Correct on first trial. **Cross Line Test II** : Failure after third trial. **Pictorial Completion Test :** 3′ 22″ ; 2 logical and 7 illogical errors ; says, " It gets me dizzy." **Tapping Test** : 87 and 82 squares respectively on first and second trial ; 2 and 1 error respectively. **School Work** : Reading : 5th-grade passage read fluently, but reproduction inaccurate. Arithmetic : Knows all fundamental processes ; makes 1 error in division.
Second Testing one day later :
Cross Line Test II : Failure on second trial. Refuses to try further. **Pictorial Completion Test** : 2′ 10″ ; 8 illogical errors. **Easy Opposites Test** : 6 errors and 1 failure ; average time 2.2″ ; range 1″ to 5″. **Kraepelin Subtraction Test :**

Subtracting 7 from 100 ; 2′ 34″, 8 errors. (Refuses to try again.) **Memory for Logical Material** — auditory verbal presentation : 7 out of 12 items given ; no attempt at logical sequence or verbal accuracy. (Attitude unfavorable.)

Third Testing one week after last testing :

Construction Test I : 26″, 8 moves. **Construction Test II** : 1′ 3″, 11 moves ; rational method. **Cross Line Test II** : Correct on first trial. **Pictorial Completion Test** : 5′ 24″ ; 1 logical and 6 illogical errors. **Easy Opposites Test** (new list used): 3 errors and 2 failures ; average time 3″.

Case 39. ———. 11 years, 6 months.

First Testing :

Binet grade : 6⅗ years. **Introductory Test** : 2′ 50″; trial and error method on triangles. **Construction Test I** : Failure ; entirely irrational procedure. **Memory for Logical Material** — visual verbal presentation : Only 2 of 20 items given. **School Work** : Reading : Simple 2nd-grade passage read slowly, but understandingly ; reproduction fair. Writing and Spelling : Writes plainly his own name and a few simple words. Arithmetic : Makes simple combinations by counting on his fingers, but often errors. Fails to make simple change and to add a few coins correctly.

Second Testing one year and eight months later :

Binet grade : 7⅖ years. **Introductory Test** : 1′ 15″; 20″ on triangles. **Construction Test I** : 12″, 8 moves. **Construction Test II** : Failure. **Puzzle Box** : Failure. **Cross Line Test I** : Failure on fourth trial. **Arbitrary Association Learning Test** : 5 errors. **Auditory Memory Span** : 4 numerals correct. **Visual Memory Span** : 5 numerals correct. **Memory for Logical Material** — visual verbal presentation : 9 of 20 items given. **Memory for Logical Material** — auditory verbal presentation : 5 of 12 items given. **School Work** : Reading, 3rd-grade passage read fluently. Reproduction poor. Writing and Spelling : Writes fairly ; spelling fair for simple words. Arithmetic : Fails to add anything except the simplest combinations ; fails to make simple change, or to add small coins correctly.

Case 40. MARTIN T. 16 years.

Binet grade : 10 years plus 2½ tests. (?) Failures : 10 years, ½ of (2), (3), and (4) ; but all 12 years correct. **Construction Test I** : 10″, 7 moves. **Construction Test II** : 1′ 33″, 16 moves. **Cross Line Test II** : Correct on third trial. **Pictorial Completion Test** : 4′ 16″, 6 illogical errors. (Retested next day : 2′ 5″, 6 illogical errors.) **Easy Opposites Test** : 4 errors and 1 failure ; average time 2.5″. **Kraepelin Subtraction Test** : Subtracting 6 from 100, time (?), 2 errors ; subtracting 4 from 100, 1′ 13″, 4 errors. **School Work** : Reading : 3rd-grade passage read stumblingly; reproduction fairly good. Writing and Spelling : Writes from dictation " The parer mad som cars " (The printer made some cards). Arithmetic : Adds, subtracts, and multiplies correctly. Cannot do long division. Makes change correctly, *e.g.*, $2.00 − $1.47 = 53¢. Oral problems done promptly, *e.g.*, 8 pairs of shoes at $1.50 a pair = $12.00. If you had some apples and gave away ½ and lost ½ of those left and then had 4, how many did you have at first?

Case 41. WILHELMINA T. 18 years.

Introductory Test : 1′ 50″. **Construction Test I** : Failure ; correct only after 5′ 15″ and 43 moves. **Construction Test II** : 5′ 30″, 48 moves. **Puzzle Box** : Failure ; in 3′ only 3 moves made ; very stupid performance. **Tapping Test** : 75 and 90 squares respectively on first and second trial ; 1 and 0 errors respectively. **Cross Line Test I** : Much difficulty in grasping idea of test ; used as practice test. **Cross Line Test II** : Failure on fourth trial. **Arbitrary Association Test** : 3 errors ; slowly done. **Easy Opposites Test** : No error or failure ; average time 1.8″. **Visual Memory — reproduction of Binet figures** : One figure correct ; the other failure. **School Work** : Reading : 5th-grade passage read fluently, with good expression. Writing and Spelling : Writes from dictation " The printer made some cards." Arithmetic : Does long division correctly ; fails on fractions.

Case 42. CATHERINE L. 16 years, 1 month.

Binet grade : 8⅕ years. Failures : 8 years, (2) and (4) ; 9 years, (2) and (4) ; 10 years, all tests. **Construction Test I** : Failure ; correct only after 6′ 37″ with 58 moves. **Construction Test II** : Correct only in 6′ 10″ with 64 moves. **Cross Line Test I** : Failure on fourth trial. **Pictorial Completion Test** : 8′ 18″, 5 illogical errors ; many absurdities.

Second Testing two months later :

Construction Test I : 6″, 7 moves. (Evidently remembered solution.) **Construction Test II** : 41″, 15 moves. (Evidently remembered solution.) **Cross Line Test I** : Does not grasp idea. **Pictorial Completion Test** : 2′ 56″, 1 logical and 5 illogical errors. **Arbitrary Association Test** : Cannot copy numbers. **Tapping Test** : 50 and 54 squares respectively on first and second trial ; 1 error each trial. **School Work** : Cannot read. **Writing and Spelling** : Cannot write. **Arithmetic** : 4 + 6 + 3 + 2 = ? Adds slowly by ones, but cannot write down the total.

Third Testing one week later (with interpreter) :

Binet grade : 9⅗ years. Failures : 8 years, (4) ; 9 years, (4) ; 10 years, (2), (3), and (4) ; 12 years, (4) and (5). **Visual Memory — reproduction of Binet figures** : Failure. **School Work** : **Arithmetic** : Cannot make change, except simplest problems, e.g., 25 ¢ − 4 ¢ = 21 ¢, but 50 ¢ − 37 ¢ = ?

Case 43. BERNARD G. 17 years, 8 months.

Binet grade : 9⅗ years. Failures : 9 years, (4) ; 10 years, (1), (3), (4) ; 12 years, (3), (4), and (5). **Introductory Test** : 1′ ; no difficulty on triangles. **Construction Test I** : 10″, 5 moves. Remarkably good record. **Construction Test II** : 41″, 12 moves. Likewise extremely good record. **Puzzle Box** : Failure. **Instructions Box** : Correct on third trial. On previous trials error only on dial. **Tapping Test** : 98 and 92 squares, respectively, first and second trial ; 2 and 1 error respectively. **Cross Line Test I** : Correct on third trial. **Cross Line Test II** : Failure on fourth trial. **Pictorial Completion Test** : 3′, 2 logical and 1 illogical error. **Easy Opposites Test** : 8 errors and 2 failures ; average time 3.5″.

Arbitrary Association Test : 3 errors.   School Work : Fails on multiplication and division.

Case 44. LEO N.   16 years, 6 months.
No records given; present standard procedure not used.

Case 45. JAMES C.   11 years.
Binet grade : 8⅗ years.   Failures : 9 years, (2) and (4) ; 10 years, all failures.   **Introductory Test** : 3′ 28″.   Construction Test I : 17″, 7 moves.   Construction Test II : Failure at end of 10′.   **Puzzle Box** : Failure at end of 6′, during which time no single correct move was made.   **Cross Line Test I** : Failure on fourth trial.   Cross Line Test II : Failure on fourth trial.   **Easy Opposites Test** : 8 failures ; average time 2.9″.   (2 failures possibly due to lack of knowledge.)   **School Work** : Reading : 3rd-grade passage read well ; reproduction accurate but somewhat meager.   Writing and Spelling : Writes from dictation " The cat ran away ", " The printer — some cards."   Writes simple stories, misspelling only unfamiliar words.   Very much better results than on performance tests.   Arithmetic : Adds correctly ; knows multiplication tables through 3's.

: **Case 46.** FREDERICK J.   13 years, 9 months.
Introductory Test : 1′ 40″.   Construction Test I : 17″, 7 moves.   Construction Test II : 1′ 59″, 19 moves.   **Puzzle Box** : 4′ 41″, 5 errors.   Instructions Box : Correct on second trial.   Cross Line Test I : Failure on fourth trial.   Cross Line Test II : Failure on fourth trial.   School Work : Reading : Cannot read 1st-grade passage.   Writing and Spelling : Cannot write any words.   **Arithmetic** : Adds, subtracts, and multiplies correctly.   Solves correctly examples such as, 2568 × 396.
Second Testing 2 years and 5 months later :
Binet grade : Through 10 years.   Failures : 9 years, (2) ; 10 years, (2) and (5) ; 12 years, (2) and (5).   **School Work** : Writes from dictation " The primo sat ctame " (The printer made some cards).   Arithmetic : Multiplies and divides correctly.

INDEX

265